When Killing Is Wrong

Shannon
mcalister

When Killing Is Wrong

Physician-Assisted Suicide and the Courts

Arthur J. Dyck

THE
PILGRIM
PRESS
Cleveland

The Pilgrim Press, Cleveland, Ohio 44115
www.pilgrimpress.com

Printed in the United States of America on acid-free paper

06 05 04 03 02 01   5 4 3 2 1

Library of Congress Cataloging-in-Publication Data
Dyck, Arthur J., 1932-
    When killing is wrong : physician-assisted suicide and the courts /
Arthur J. Dyck.
       p. cm.
    Includes bibliographical references and index.
    ISBN 0-8298-1417-5 (pbk. : alk. paper)
    1. Assisted suicide – Law and legislation – United States. 2. Assisted
suicide – Moral and ethical aspects – United States   I. Title.

KF3827.E87 D93 2001
174′.24 – dc21
                                   2001021103

Contents

Preface

WITH REGARD TO PHYSICIAN-ASSISTED SUICIDE, there is a serious conflict in American courts. To be sure, this conflict is one of differing ways of interpreting the Constitution of the United States. But that aspect of the conflict is not the focus of this book. Rather, the concern of this book is that the federal court opinions on physician-assisted suicide (hereafter PAS) exhibit two very divergent views of when it is that killing is morally and legally wrong. If those in the courts who advocate a constitutional right to PAS were to prevail, the very basis of homicide law would be radically altered. The traditions that shaped more than seven hundred years of Anglo-American law would be suppressed in favor of a quite different moral, and philosophical or theological, tradition. The current synthesis of concepts derived from Jewish and Christian sources and from the natural rights tradition originating with Hobbes and Locke would largely, if not completely, be replaced by a tradition forged from certain aspects of the thinking of John Stuart Mill. This particular, rather truncated version of Mill, as this book will argue, does not by itself provide a principled moral and legal basis for homicide law, and certainly not for the prevention of suicide and assisting in it.

But has not the United States Supreme Court effectively ended this conflict in 1997 by issuing its unanimous decisions denying that there is a constitutional right to PAS? (See *Washington v. Glucksberg* and *Vacco v. Quill.*) No, it has not. For one thing, there are clearly judges who favor such a right. One need look no further than the judges upholding the opinions of the Ninth Circuit Court of Appeals in *Compassion in Dying v. State of Washington* (1996) and the Second Circuit Court of Appeals in *Quill v. Vacco* (1996), the very court decisions overturned by the Supreme Court in 1997. The composition of the Supreme Court will, of course, change over time, with the prospect that future decisions regarding PAS could change as well. But secondly, the issue of what makes killing wrong, when it is, and what moral and legal concepts will provide a principled basis for homicide law remains unresolved. Why is that?

In the opinion Chief Justice William Rehnquist wrote for the Supreme Court in 1997, he appeals to facts and law. For his arguments he draws upon arguments contained in previous court opinions. Legally, he is quite appropriately appealing to precedent. From a philosophical perspective, however, this constitutes an appeal to authority, an appeal that does not offer a philosophical justification for the arguments and court opinions he cites. By contrast, the opinions exhibiting the tradition drawn from Mill go beyond facts and legal precedents by resorting to philosophical modes of argumentation and by making unexamined assumptions about human nature at odds with what has been assumed by many previous courts, as cited by Rehnquist. This has the effect of leaving the arguments of the Supreme Court without a current philosophical underpinning, while those who favor PAS have provided current philosophical arguments, albeit not always explicitly, for their position. Since, in my view, the version of Mill now found in the American courts would leave homicide law without a principled basis, there is an urgent need to examine carefully what philosophical justification exists for the principles that now guide and support homicide law. This book intends to provide such a justification.

Given the conflict that now divides American jurists and court opinions, this book will identify the contrasting views as to when it is that killing is wrong. This will entail a careful examination of the concepts and traditions that shape these conflicting ways of thinking about killing and homicide law. The book will elicit and render explicit the moral framework that undergirds homicide law as understood in the Supreme Court opinion of 1997. That framework will be defended philosophically. That defense will, at the same time, be a defense of laws that prohibit anyone from assisting in a suicide.

Furthermore, the version of Mill now found in the courts does not square with Mill's thinking seen from a more comprehensive perspective. Mill was concerned that the rules that are essential to individual security and communal life be upheld and enforced. Hence, at the conclusion of the book, I will argue there is no need to suppress other traditions now in synthesis by invoking the Millian tradition. The philosophy of Mill can be synthesized with the traditions of Jewish, Christian, Hobbesian, and Lockean origins. That does not, I think, require a resolution of some of the contrasting reflections regarding human nature that are to be found in these rich and, in a number of ways, quite varied traditions.

Since this book is concerned to cherish and protect human life, it is fitting that I first acknowledge Joseph R. Stanton and his wife, Mary. The late Dr. Stanton, though suffering from the crippling and painful effects of polio, was tireless in his efforts to promote the utmost respect for life. He first alerted me to the trends within the courts on matters of life and death, making certain that I had copies of these decisions without delay. Joseph and Mary shared in this work of educating many; I was far from the lone benefactor of their labor. The late Paul Ramsey also taught me a great deal about the moral reasoning of the courts, beginning with the Quinlan case in 1976. I am deeply grateful for the stimulation, assistance, and insights of all three of these admirable individuals.

I must pay tribute to my esteemed colleagues Stanley J. Reiser and the late William J. Curran. It was Stanley, the physician, who had the idea that I should address matters ethical arising within the practice of medicine; it was William, the lawyer, whose editorials and conversations taught me much about how the law and medicine intersect. I cherish deeply all I learned from them as we taught medical ethics together for a number of years. I now enjoy collegial instruction from Judith Kinley, a nurse, and the physician Richard Norton, as we continue to offer a course in ethics within medical practice. I am profoundly grateful to all four of these splendid, devoted teachers for enriching me intellectually, morally, and spiritually for tasks I neither could, nor should, undertake without such enrichment.

I am thankful for the helpful responses I have had from so many students. In particular, I have enjoyed valuable material as well as intellectual assistance from Karey Harwood, Gretchen Landwehr, and Nancy Platteborze. Nancy should be singled out for helping me clarify some of the issues raised in the book. Greg Ingram made some excellent editorial suggestions. All of these students were a source of encouragement. Arnold Reif has sent me numerous articles.

Everyone should know a bright, witty, and intellectually engaging minister. I am fortunate to have had many a lively conversation with Joe Bassett, pastor of the First Church in Chestnut Hill, Massachusetts. My gratitude is far deeper than I can convey by these few words.

Everyone should have superb secretarial assistance. I have it! Kay Shanahan is simply the best!

I do want to thank Richard Brown, who first, so enthusiastically, accepted the idea of this book and urged me to sign up with the Pilgrim Press. Thanks also to George R. Graham, present academic book editor of Pilgrim, for timely editorial suggestions I gladly accepted. I am grateful as well to John Eagleson for his superb work as a copy editor.

1

Divisions over
Physician-Assisted Suicide

O N JUNE 26, 1997, the United States Supreme Court announced
its unanimous decisions to uphold the constitutionality of the
laws prohibiting assisted suicide in the states of Washington and
New York.[1] These decisions denied the claims of the Ninth and Second Courts of Appeals that there is a constitutional right to PAS.[2]
These decisions by the Supreme Court and claims by the courts of
appeals represented conflicting legal traditions and modes of moral
argumentation. In order to advance the debate over assisted suicide,
these divergent traditions need to be brought into a synthesis. By
considering recent cases about assisted suicide and the legal concepts behind them, this book will establish a synthesis from the
primary legal traditions about the issue of assisted suicide that undergirds the dignity of human life and lends further support to the
1997 Supreme Court decision against legalizing assisted suicide.

Writing for the Supreme Court in 1997, Chief Justice Rehnquist
found no constitutionally protected "right to commit suicide which
itself includes a right to assistance in doing so."[3] Indeed, "for over
700 years Anglo-American common law tradition has punished
or otherwise disapproved of both suicide and assisting suicide."[4]
Furthermore, he noted that the great majority of states have laws
explicitly prohibiting assistance in a suicide; at the time of this de-

---

1. *Washington v. Glucksberg,* 117 S.Ct. 2258 (1997); *Vacco v. Quill* 117 S.Ct.
2293 (1997).
2. *Compassion in Dying v. State of Washington,* 79 F. 3rd 790 (9th Cir. 1996);
Quill v. Vacco, 80 F. 3rd 716 (2nd Cir. 1996).
3. *Washington v. Glucksberg,* 2269.
4. Ibid., 2263.

cision, nineteen states had defeated one or more recent attempts to pass legislation that would have permitted PAS.[5]

For now, then, the prohibition of assisted suicide, found in common law and existing legislation, remains intact. But what of the foreseeable future? The possibility of enacting state laws permitting PAS in particular circumstances was not expressly ruled out. For one thing, the justices agreed that the states should be free to evaluate the area of PAS. In her concurring opinion, Justice Sandra Day O'Connor expressed this point as follows:

> As the Court recognizes, states are presently undertaking extensive and serious evaluation of physician assisted suicide. . . . In such circumstances, "the challenging task of crafting appropriate procedures for safeguarding liberty interests is entrusted to the laboratory of the States . . . in the first instance."[6]

This understanding of the responsibilities of the states leaves open the possibility that laws favoring PAS could be enacted. Such laws, in turn, could, if challenged and accepted for review, come under the scrutiny of the Supreme Court. Moreover, the concurring opinions of Justices Breyer, Souter, and Stevens particularly, can be read to suggest that, given the right case, these justices might find a carefully, narrowly tailored law favoring PAS constitutionally sound; at the same time, these same justices might find a particular law banning assisted suicide unconstitutional. However these justices and the other members of the Court might vote on a specific state law pertaining to assisted suicide, it is the case that there are important differences among the existing members of the Court with respect to their approaches to assisted suicide and the issues raised by it. These differences are such that the composition of the Court will be critical for determining what policies regarding PAS will prevail in the United States, whether in the near or more distant future. Certainly, the Supreme Court would have declared a constitutional right to PAS if a majority of its members had shared the moral and legal reasoning of those who affirmed such a right in the Ninth and Second Circuit Courts of Appeals.

Efforts to pass legislation permitting PAS can be expected to continue. The conflicting modes of thinking identifiable in the Supreme

---

5. Ibid.
6. Ibid., 2303.

Court and other federal courts exist in a very evenly divided American populace judging by the voting on recent state referenda designed to legalize PAS. In Washington and California voters defeated such referenda by a 54 percent majority; in Oregon's first vote on such a referendum, it was approved by 51 percent of those voting, representing 34 percent of registered voters.[7] These votes reflect situations in which a determined minority of opponents or proponents of PAS can tip the balance in favor of their views either by influencing legislation or by bringing a compelling case before the Supreme Court. Indeed, Oregon's referendum favoring PAS became law after the Supreme Court's decision in 1997.[8]

How important are the issues that divide the courts and populace over whether PAS should be legally permissible in some circumstances? A major clue that the outcome of the debate over PAS is momentous and far-reaching in its implications for American law and social policy has already been provided: for over seven hundred years, Anglo-American law has opposed PAS. One can well suspect that a particular way of thinking is behind this opposition, dominant enough to hold sway for all those years. If, then, a substitute for that way of thinking is being sought, as it is by some, it is important to assess whether such a change provides a basis for sustaining communal life and its legal structure.

The question being raised about the sustainability of a way of thinking is actually a twofold question: first, is opposition to assisted suicide rooted in a view of morality and law that is essential to sustaining communal life because it provides the kind and degree of moral and legal protection of individual life and liberty necessary for perpetuating communal life at all? Secondly, is the affirmation of assisted suicide rooted in a view such that its implementation in law and social policy would undermine the protection of individual life and liberty necessary to perpetuating communal life? But the fact that a traditional way of thinking is seven hundred years old and finds expression in contemporary law and policy does not by itself justify its dominance or even its continuation. Even if it is a way of thinking that offers a sustainable basis for forming and maintaining communal life, a substitute for such a way of thinking

---

7. Initiative for Death with Dignity, Washington Initiative No. 19 (1991); The California Death with Dignity Act; California Proposition No. 161 (1992); Death with Dignity Act, Oregon, Measure 16 (1994).

8. Oregon Revised Statutes, 1996 Supplement 127.800–127.897.

could be defended if adopting it would also maintain rather than undermine what makes communal life possible while at the same time expanding rights in new ways. It is no wonder that the debate over PAS can arouse such deep emotions. Not only does this debate confront us with human suffering and difficult choices about how to respond to it, but the debate entails and exhibits conflicting ways of thinking about the moral and legal bases essential for sustaining individual and communal life.

There are no less than three different ways of thinking that vie for ascendancy in American courts. I am going to call these ways of thinking "traditions." These ways of thinking each fit the dictionary definition of a tradition as "an inherited, established or customary pattern of thought."[9] Actually, these patterns of thought are "inherited" in the sense of being present for more than a generation; "established" in the sense of providing a rationale, often implicitly, for individual institutional and legal decisions; and "customary" in the sense of finding expression in conventional societal practices and individual action, often unwittingly.

All three traditions have different historical roots but all have persisted in shaping court opinions. The first and oldest tradition is rooted in Judaism and Christianity; the second in Thomas Hobbes; and the third in John Stuart Mill.[10] As Max Stackhouse has carefully documented, the first two traditions achieved what he calls the "Liberal-Puritan Synthesis."[11] Together these traditions still provide a rationale for modern Western democratic institutions and practices. The Hobbesian outlook, designated as 'liberal" by Stackhouse, views natural, inalienable rights as rationally self-evident; Puritans viewed these same rights as divinely and rationally revealed truths. Stackhouse further claims that this synthesis, almost imperceptibly, has largely been replaced by appeals to utility as a basis for justifying policy, shaped by the heritage of Mill.

The synthesis described by Stackhouse is evident in the American Declaration of Independence. To say that individuals are "born equal" is to take the view shared by Judaism and Christianity that

9. *Webster's Tenth New Collegiate Dictionary.*
10. The tradition rooted in Hobbes includes John Locke as well; that of Mill includes Bentham; and the tradition developing from Judaism and Christianity has many philosophical representatives, most notably W. D. Ross in the twentieth century. See *The Right and the Good* (Oxford: Oxford University Press, 1930).
11. Max Stackhouse, *Creeds, Society, and Human Rights: A Study in Three Cultures* (Grand Rapids, Mich.: Eerdmans, 1984).

all human beings are children of God, created in the image of God, a view that helped defeat the practice of slavery.[12] But instead of speaking of "the law written on the heart," the language becomes Hobbesian: Human beings are said to be endowed by their Creator with inalienable *rights* to life, liberty, and the pursuit of happiness. Human beings are equals with respect to possessing these natural rights of sacred origin. This combination of the two traditions is definitely present in court cases concerned with the withdrawal of life-sustaining treatment from those who are deemed seriously and irreversibly ill.[13] And, as our analysis of the Supreme Court decisions regarding PAS will amply reveal, these two traditions have combined to shape current laws against assisted suicide.

With regard to the right to life, the terms that emerge refer to this right as both "sacred" and "inalienable." Both of these terms describe the right to life as "naturally" belonging to human beings and thus a right that can neither be taken away nor given away. As it occurs in legal reasoning, the convergence of Puritan and liberal thought is around the conception of a natural right, a permanent possession of every human being. For purposes of this book, I will refer to what Stackhouse called the "Liberal-Puritan Synthesis" as the "Natural Rights Synthesis."

With respect to the Natural Rights Synthesis, the Millian tradition as it now appears in the courts represents a significant departure. A particular version of the Millian tradition has emerged strongly in the court decisions concerned with PAS as well as those concerned with the withdrawal of life-sustaining treatment. This tradition began earlier in American law and its influence pervades law in a number of areas.[14] Its presence in what the media tends to call "right to die" cases is a very critical development because it signals a change in how rights are understood, the right to life in particular. That change in thinking about life as a moral and legal right is not one that can be integrated into, or harmonized with, the

---

12. See David Brion Davis, *The Problem of Slavery in Western Culture* (Ithaca, N.Y.: Cornell University Press, 1966).

13. All three traditions are clearly represented in the case of *Brophy v. New England Sinai Hospital,* 497 N.E. 2nd 626 (1986). The analysis of this case is found in Arthur J. Dyck, *Rethinking Rights and Responsibilities: The Moral Bonds of Community* (Cleveland: Pilgrim Press, 1994), 278–85.

14. For a discussion of this particular version of Mill in American law, see Mary Ann Glendon, *Rights Talk: The Impoverishment of Political Discourse* (New York: Free Press, 1991).

Natural Rights Synthesis. The change can be traced, to begin with, to Jeremy Bentham.

Bentham, taking aim at the French Declaration of Rights, issued his own declaration: "*Natural rights* is simple nonsense: natural and imprescriptible rights, rhetorical nonsense—nonsense upon stilts. There is no right that, when the abolition of it is advantageous to society, should not be abolished."[15] Mill retains this view of rights. Rights are what justice requires. As Mill puts it, "Justice implies something that is not only right to do and wrong not to do but that some person can claim from us as his moral right."[16] But Mill does not supply us with a list of what justice requires. Rights are to be judged by what results in utility, the greatest happiness for the greatest number. The individual right to equality requires each person's happiness to count as one in calculating the greatest happiness for the greatest number. But, for Mill, equality as a right is qualified as follows: "All persons are deemed to have a right to equality of treatment, except when some recognized social expediency requires the reverse."[17] Human beings are not born equal in Mill's view, but are equal insofar as it serves to maximize utility. Governments calculate this right and others in accord with social expediency.

Mill regards the right to liberty as one that requires special protection so as not to be unduly encroached upon by governments. In one of its expressions, it should be regarded as absolute. As Mill expresses it: "The only part of the conduct of anyone for which he is amenable to society is that which concerns others. In the part which merely concerns himself, over his own body and mind, the individual is sovereign."[18] In a further elaboration of this right to liberty, Mill adds that each individual "is the proper guardian of his own health, whether bodily, or mental or spiritual."[19] To protect this individual liberty, Mill enunciates the following principle:

> The only purpose for which power can be rightfully exercised over any member of a civilized community, against his will, is to prevent harm to others. His own good, either physical

---

15. Jeremy Bentham, "Anarchical Fallacies," in *Society, Law, and Morality,* ed. Frederick A. Olafson (Englewood Cliffs, N.J.: Prentice-Hall, 1961), 347.
16. John Stuart Mill, "Utilitarianism," in *The Philosophy of John Stuart Mill,* ed. Marshall Cohen (New York: Random House, 1961), 380.
17. Ibid., 396.
18. "On Liberty," in ibid., 197.
19. Ibid., 200.

or moral, is not a sufficient warrant. He cannot rightfully be compelled to do or to forebear because it will be better for him to do so, because it would make him happier, because in the opinions of others, to do so would be wise, or even right.[20]

This principle is one that we find applied in American courts. In a decision by the Massachusetts Supreme Judicial Court this very quotation from Mill was cited to justify an individual's alleged wish to die by the removal of nutrition and hydration.[21] This same principle was at the core of the reasoning used by the Ninth Circuit Court of Appeals to argue that PAS is a constitutionally protected right.

To begin with, then, the Ninth Circuit Court of Appeals argued that individuals, as sovereigns over their own bodies, already have a constitutionally protected right to refuse treatment in situations that hasten death. Choosing PAS when terminally ill is, like refusing life-sustaining treatment, a personal decision that should not be forbidden by law. Furthermore, employing a mode of reasoning also found in Mill, the Ninth Circuit Court argued that refusing life-sustaining treatment, such as artificially administered nutrition and hydration, has the same effect as PAS: both hasten death. Therefore, the Ninth Circuit Court concluded, these decisions do not differ significantly morally and, hence, should not differ legally: both the right to refuse life-sustaining treatment and the right to PAS should be constitutionally protected rights. The Ninth Circuit Court was fully aware that its majority opinion drew on Millian principles.[22] From the standpoint of the Ninth Circuit Court, under certain circumstances a request for PAS is as reasonable as a request to be free of life-sustaining medical interventions.

From a Hobbesian perspective, the whole idea that committing suicide is sometimes a rational decision is fundamentally mistaken. Human beings naturally seek to preserve their own lives. Any desire or decision to destroy one's own life is irrational. Indeed, courts do speak of suicide as irrational self-destruction and hence an action to try to prevent rather than assist.[23] Suicide, as an irrational ac-

---

20. Ibid., 197.
21. *Brophy v. New England Sinai Hospital.*
22. *Compassion in Dying v. State of Washington* 79 F. 3rd 790 (9th Cir. 1996), footnote, 124, 833–34. In this footnote, Judge Reinhardt accepts the use of principles drawn from Mill, but not Judge Posner's willingness to have PAS legislated in the states.
23. *Brophy v. New England Sinai Hospital,* Lynch, J., dissenting.

tion once uniformly regarded as one of the criteria for diagnosing a state of depression, is not to be punished as such, but assisting someone to commit suicide should be.[24] The right to life, according to Hobbes, is ours by our very nature; it is not something we should ever bargain away or compromise in the social contract that legitimates sovereignty. We can, and should, give up some of our liberty, but not our right to life. The legitimacy of sovereignty is based on its actual power to protect life. This is true because human beings naturally seek pleasure and avoid pain for themselves and their desires put them in life-threatening competition for goods, unless protected by the coercive power of a sovereign.[25]

Hobbes bases his assertion of the right to life on his doctrine of human nature, his theological anthropology: human beings naturally seek to preserve their own lives; no government edict can or should seek to change that reality. Whereas Mill also portrayed human beings as naturally seeking pleasure and avoiding pain for themselves, he did not explicitly call attention to a natural desire to preserve one's own life. This difference between the theological anthropologies of Hobbes and Mill has a very significant effect on how one approaches the possibility of morally and legally justifying assisted suicide. Mill's view of human nature allows for a rational desire to end one's life and to relinquish voluntarily one's right to life. After all, in a situation that an individual may perceive as devoid of pleasure and the future prospect of pleasure and as presently and foreseeably exceedingly painful, a decision to end one's life could indeed appear, to such an individual and to others, to be reasonable. According to the Hobbesian conception of human nature, it is contrary to our nature to seek to relinquish one's right to life and irrational to destroy one's life.

The Puritans, however, could ally themselves with the Hobbesian conception of a natural right to life without accepting the Hobbesian view of human nature. After all, their understanding of the biblical notion of the law written on the heart clearly forbade killing, oneself or others. This was a law of nature, and so the claim, the right, to have one's life protected would be in accord with this natural moral law. However, this means that human beings by

---

24. See Thomas Marzen et al., "Suicide: A Constitutional Right?" *Duquesne Law Review* 24, no. 1 (1985): 1–242.

25. Thomas Hobbes, *Leviathan* (1651; reprint, Indianapolis: Bobbs-Merrill, 1958), chapters 13 and 17.

nature are not only prone to seek pleasure for themselves and to vie with others in harmful ways, but also as creatures of God prone to have some desire and knowledge to live in accord with the moral law.[26] Given the ability to know right from wrong and given also the egoistic strivings that threaten individual and communal life, democratic institutions are at once possible and necessary.[27] The Puritans had a social conception of human nature, rather than the egoistic, individualistic conceptions shared by Hobbes and Mill. Nevertheless, since the Puritans and Hobbesians both had solid reasons to affirm the right to life as natural and inalienable, the differences in their theological anthropologies did not explicitly enter into the deliberations regarding homicide law in American courts, certainly not in the decisions cited by the Supreme Court's unanimous rejection of a constitutional right to PAS.

But the particular version of Mill present in the majority opinion of the Ninth Circuit Court does rest in part upon an implicit theological anthropology that does not, as such, provide a basis for retaining the Natural Rights Synthesis and its affirmation of the right to life as natural and inalienable. And, interestingly enough, as we shall see, the Ninth Circuit Court depicts opposition to a constitutional right to PAS as largely religious. At the same time, the Court's view is portrayed as morally and religiously neutral. Does this mean that the debate over PAS as a legal or constitutional right has to involve a debate over which theological anthropology should form the basis for homicide law in general, and the laws on assisted suicide and euthanasia in particular? Although the theological premises of the debate over PAS and euthanasia should be identified for reasons that will later become evident, one major purpose of this book is to indicate the grounds on which theological conflicts can and should be avoided in the deliberations over PAS and euthanasia in the courts and legislative bodies.

Another major purpose of this book is to identify the special version of Mill present in the decisions of the Ninth and Second Circuit Courts of Appeals. Identifying this version of Mill will reveal just how extensively it suppresses the traditions that underlie and shape the Natural Rights Synthesis embedded in past and present

---

26. A common biblical source for this is in Romans, chapter 2.
27. See this point in a discussion of the contributions of Calvin and Calvinism to modern democracy in Dyck, *Rethinking Rights and Responsibilities*, 244–47.

homicide law and constitutional decisions regarding it. This, I will argue, is problematic because the traditions being suppressed serve to uphold certain responsibilities and rights that should be regarded as requisites of individual and communal life and that should be taught and enforced by law. I will argue that the decisions of the Ninth and Second Circuit Courts would, if adopted, in principle and in practice, undermine these requisites of individual and communal life and the laws now protecting them. But rejecting the special version of Mill in these courts does not, I will try to show, mean that the Millian tradition as a whole needs to be suppressed. There are elements in Mill that are aimed at supporting these requisites, and if attended to, could forge a new synthesis properly protective of individual life. Such a new synthesis would not permit PAS and euthanasia. At the same time, it would and should energize efforts to keep increasing, as we are, the technical ability to relieve pain and to incorporate this knowledge into medical education and routine medical practice. These purposes are pursued in the three chapters that follow.

In chapter 2, I will examine the conflicts between the special version of Mill found in the Ninth and Second Circuit Courts of Appeals and the reasoning typical of other traditions contained in constitutional law as described by the Supreme Court in its respective decisions on PAS. The central conflict described in that chapter, that is, whether PAS differs morally in any significant way from comfort-only care, is a conflict over what makes killing wrong when it is wrong.

Chapter 3 takes up this conflict over what makes killing wrong when it is wrong. This it does by comparing the reasoning of the Ninth Circuit with the reasoning of the Supreme Court as expressed in the opinions written by Judge Reinhardt and Chief Justice Rehnquist respectively. The chapter further identifies the differences between the special version of Mill espoused by Judge Reinhardt and the Natural Rights Synthesis as embedded in the laws and court decisions cited by Chief Justice Rehnquist. The chapter ends by revealing what it is that Judge Reinhardt omits of Mill's thinking and by suggesting reasons for developing a new synthesis incorporating Mill into the existing Natural Rights Synthesis and what it stands for.

What I will be arguing in the fourth and concluding chapter is that: (1) there is a moral structure that supports Chief Justice Rehnquist's portrayal of what is harmful about the act of killing and assisting someone to commit such an act, including the act of killing oneself; (2) this moral structure would be threatened or undermined by legalizing PAS; (3) there are elements in Mill's thinking that lend support to the preceding two contentions. If jurists were to work with these elements in Mill's thinking, they would, I contend, accomplish two things: (1) forge and work with a new synthesis of the three major traditions now shaping American law; and (2) avoid the theological conflicts now implicitly engendered by certain assumptions about human nature implicit in the special version of Mill now current in American law.

2

Conflicting Modes of Moral Argumentation

O N MARCH 6, 1996, the Ninth Circuit Court of Appeals in California held that there is a constitutionally protected right to PAS; on April 2, less than a month later, the Second Court of Appeals did so as well.[1] As we have noted, these are the two decisions that the United States Supreme Court reversed on June 26, 1997. These decisions and their subsequent reversals point to a fundamental conflict about the modes of moral argumentation used in the courts.

Ninth Circuit Judge Reinhardt, who wrote that court's majority opinion, accepted by a vote of eight to three, anticipated strong opposition. Indeed, he anticipated one of the very arguments that united the Supreme Court against his ruling when he wrote:

> To those who argue that courts should refrain from declaring that the terminally ill have a constitutional right to physician-assisted suicide and that we should leave such matters to the individual states, we reply that where important liberty interests are at stake it is not the proper role of the state to adopt statutes totally prohibiting their exercise.[2]

In his dissenting opinion, Ninth Circuit Judge Kleinfeld explicitly attacked this argument:

> That a question is important does not imply that it is constitutional. The Founding Fathers did not establish the United

---

1. *Compassion in Dying v. State of Washington*, 79 F. 3rd 790 (9th Cir. 1996); *Quill v. Vacco*, 80 F. 3rd 716 (2nd Cir. 1996).
2. *Compassion in Dying v. State of Washington* (1996), 833.

States as a democratic republic so that elected officials would decide trivia, while all great questions would be decided by the judiciary.[3]

Still other members of the Ninth Circuit Court strongly believed that this decision exceeded the powers of the judiciary and called for a vote to rehear the case. The vote to rehear was lost. Writing in dissent of that vote against rehearing, Circuit Judge O'Scanlain, joined by Circuit Judges Trott and Kleinfeld, minced no words on the issue of judicial authority, calling the decision "a shockingly broad act of judicial legislation"[4] and challenging its merits on the grounds that:

> ...the opinion usurps the state legislative function, and in doing so silences the voice of the people of Washington and defies the Supreme Court's call for judicial restraint in the area of substantive due process.... The Supreme Court has never recognized a substantive due process right without first finding that there is a tradition of protecting that particular interest. Here, there is absolutely no tradition of protecting that particular interest. Almost all states forbid assisted suicide and some states even permit the use of nondeadly force to thwart suicide attempts. No state has ever accepted consent of the victim as a defense to a charge of homicide. These are political judgments made by the democratic process; if they are no longer "politically correct," let the legislatures act to change them, not life-tenured judges immune from the voters' reach.[5]

As we shall see, the Supreme Court sided with the dissenters, making these very points as well. Judge Reinhardt tried to blunt this kind of criticism in yet another way when he wrote:

> We also recognize that other able and dedicated jurists, construing the Constitution as they believe it must be construed, may disagree not only with the result we reach but with our method of constitutional analysis. Given the nature of the judicial process and the complexity of the task of determining the rights and interests comprehended by the Constitution, good

---

3. Ibid., Kleinfeld, J., dissenting, 858.
4. *Compassion in Dying v. State of Washington*, 85 F. 3rd 1440 (9th Cir. June 12, 1996), O'Scanlain dissenting, 1442.
5. Ibid., 1444–45.

faith disagreements within the judiciary should not surprise or disturb anyone who follows the development of the law.[6]

Certainly there have been disagreements among federal judges as to how the constitution is to be interpreted, and anyone can reasonably expect that there will be such disagreements in the future. But it is not the fact that there is disagreement in the courts but the nature of certain disagreements in the Ninth Circuit that are of interest for the purposes of this book.

Judge Reinhardt claimed that his opinion was "guided by the facts and the law."[7] However, his opinion went far beyond what jurists ordinarily refer to as "the facts and the law." In fact, within the Ninth Circuit a full-fledged debate over the morality of assisted suicide took place. That debate mirrored the debate one finds in the popular and scholarly literature and drew upon that literature. Underlying that debate is an even more fundamental dispute, one not specifically addressed, but certainly exhibited in what were sometimes sharp exchanges. It is fundamental because nothing less than conflicting visions of law and morality, and of the philosophical and theological traditions shaping these visions, are at stake. Before beginning an examination of these conflicting visions and traditions, the reader needs to know something about the history of the case before this court and exactly what was decided.

Three terminally ill patients, four physicians, and Compassion in Dying, a nonprofit corporation, sought to have Washington State's law against causing or aiding another person to commit suicide declared to be in violation of the federal Constitution. Barbara J. Rothstein, chief judge of the United States District Court for the Western District of Washington, did just that.[8] The state appealed. A three-judge panel of the Ninth Circuit, by a two to one vote, reversed that decision.[9] Subsequently, the Ninth Circuit Court voted to rehear the case *en banc*. In the Ninth Circuit, that requires eleven members ruling on behalf of the whole court. There was further dissent in the Ninth Circuit that led to a vote to have all eligible members of the court hear the case since the eight judges signing

---

6. *Compassion in Dying v. State of Washington* (1996), 838.

7. Ibid., 836.

8. *Compassion in Dying v. State of Washington*, 850 F. Supp. 1454 (W.D. Wash. 1994).

9. *Compassion in Dying v. State of Washington*, No. 94-35534, 1995 WL 94679 (9th Cir. Mar. 9, 1995).

on to Judge Reinhardt's opinion constituted only one-third of the court's thirty-three eligible judges. As we have already observed, this vote to rehear was lost, but it provided some additional dissent, written in opposition to Judge Reinhardt's decision.[10] One further note: all three of the patients had died before Judge Reinhardt's ruling; two had died by the time the District Court issued its decision.[11]

What was it that the Ninth Circuit Court decided? Judge Reinhardt, writing for the majority meeting *en banc,* described its holding as follows:

> We hold that a liberty interest exists in the choice of how and when one dies, and that the provision of the Washington statute banning assisted suicide, as applied to competent, terminally ill adults who wish to hasten their deaths by obtaining medication prescribed by their doctors, violates the Due Process clause.[12]

Judge Reinhardt characterized the "liberty interest" that should be protected by the Due Process clause of the Fourteenth Amendment of the United States Constitution as a choice of "how and when one dies," not as a choice to commit suicide.[13] He offered the following explanation for this language:

> The liberty interest we examine encompasses a whole range of acts that are generally not considered to constitute "suicide." Included within the liberty interest we examine, is, for example, the act of refusing or terminating unwanted medical treatment.... The law does not classify the death of a patient that results from the granting of his wish to decline or discontinue treatment as "suicide." Nor does the law label the acts of those who help the patient carry out that wish, whether by physically disconnecting the respirator or by removing an intravenous tube, as assistance in suicide. Accordingly, we believe that the broader terms—"the right to die," "controlling the time and manner of one's death," and "hastening one's

---

10. See notes 4 and 5 above.
11. *Compassion in Dying v. State of Washington* (1996), 795.
12. Ibid., 838.
13. Similarly, Reinhardt speaks of this liberty interest as one of "determining the time and manner of one's death." Ibid., 801–2.

death"—more accurately describe the liberty interest at issue here. . . . We have serious doubts that the terms "suicide" and "assisted suicide" are appropriate legal descriptions of the specific conduct at issue here.[14]

But, lest there be any doubt about the exact nature of the "specific conduct at issue here," Judge Reinhardt took pains to emphasize what it is and how it is to be defined:

> For purposes of this opinion, we use physician-assisted suicide as it is used by the parties and district court and as it is frequently used: the prescribing of medication by a physician for the purpose of enabling a patient to end his life. [Footnote omitted] It is only that conduct that the plaintiffs urge be held constitutionally protected in this case.[15]

All of this is in an early section of Judge Reinhardt's opinion entitled "Defining the Liberty Interest and Other Relevant Terms."[16] In point of fact, this whole section and what we have quoted from it is not merely a matter of defining terms. Rather Reinhardt is also expressing a particular moral stance, namely, that for terminally ill individuals, refusing treatment that may have the effect of hastening death or compromising life is not distinguishable in any significant way from committing suicide. As the analysis below will document, this moral stance is an important step in the development of Reinhardt's argument for a constitutional right to PAS.

As we will also observe shortly, the Second Circuit Court of Appeals rests its whole case for finding New York's law banning assisted suicide unconstitutional on this very moral stance and mode of moral reasoning. Chief Justice Rehnquist, writing for a unanimous Supreme Court, rejected this moral stance and mode of moral reasoning. This conflict between differing modes of moral reasoning is the concern of this chapter. The conflicting traditions with their differing versions of morality and differing theological anthropologies will be further elaborated and analyzed in subsequent chapters.

---

14. Ibid., 802.
15. Ibid.
16. Ibid., 801–2.

DISTINGUISHING ASSISTED SUICIDE FROM REFUSAL OF LIFE-SUSTAINING TREATMENT

As indicated previously, Reinhardt characterized PAS as a liberty interest in choosing "how and when to die." This liberty interest includes actions that terminate or refuse unwanted medical treatment. In Reinhardt's view, requesting physician assistance to commit suicide and refusing and terminating medical treatment are all equally acts of hastening death. All of these actions have the same purpose, namely, to die and to do so sooner rather than later. As Reinhardt expressly indicated, "it is the end and not the means that defines the liberty interest."[17]

Reinhardt is judging purposes, intentions, and interests by their results. More importantly, as in Mill's mode of moral reasoning, he is determining whether an action is ethical by its consequences. He was very explicit on this point:

> ...we see little, if any, difference for constitutional or ethical purposes between providing medication with a double effect and providing medication with a single effect, as long as one of the known effects in each case is to hasten the end of the patient's life. Similarly, we see no ethical or constitutionally cognizable difference between a doctor's pulling the plug on a respirator and his prescribing drugs which will permit a terminally ill patient to end his own life.[18]

A physician and a patient may intend to relieve pain by increasing the dosage of drugs to be administered, but if doing so in any way hastens death, it is no different morally from hastening death by means of providing and using a known lethal dose of drugs. It is, as Reinhardt said, the end that counts, not the means. He dismissed, therefore, the position of the American Medical Association, enunciated in its amicus brief submitted to his court, because that brief sanctions the practice of administering medicine with a dual effect when done for the sake of comfort but opposes the legalization of PAS.[19]

Reinhardt admonished physicians to drop this whole appeal to a "double effect" to justify the distinction between PAS and com-

---

17. Ibid., 801.
18. Ibid., 824.
19. Ibid., Footnote 102, 828.

fort care that provides the pain relief that is intended but also results in hastening death, an unintended effect. Equating instances of refusal or withdrawal of medical treatment with PAS both ethically and constitutionally is a significant step toward recognizing a constitutional right to die that includes the right to PAS. Reinhardt interpreted the Supreme Court's decision in *Cruzan* as having accepted a constitutional right to die in a case in which Reinhardt views Nancy Cruzan's death as caused by the withdrawal of artificially administered nutrition and hydration, and not by her underlying disease.[20] Also, more than forty states, Washington included, have approved living wills or advance directives in which competent adults may declare their wishes not to be kept alive by medical treatment in the late stages of a terminal illness.[21] From Reinhardt's point of view, then, the Supreme Court and most states have in effect endorsed "hastening death" and should do so explicitly in the case of PAS by removing current laws banning assistance in a suicide.

In *Quill v. Vacco,* the Second Circuit Court of Appeals held that New York's complete ban on assisted suicide violated the Equal Protection Clause of the Fourteenth Amendment.[22] This clause demands that no state shall "deny to any person within its jurisdictions the equal protection of the laws." It was persons who wished to have their physicians assist them to commit suicide who were allegedly being denied the equal protection of the laws. How did the court reach this conclusion?

The case bears the name of Timothy Quill, one of three physicians who challenged the constitutionality of New York's ban on assisted suicide, a ban that prevented them as physicians from carrying out the requests of their patients for assistance in ending their lives.[23] Three patients, then in the final stages of terminal illness, joined their physicians in this challenge brought in the United States District Court for the Southern District of New York. These patients then alleged that they were terminally ill, with no prospect of recovery, seeking the assistance of a physician to hasten death, certainly and humanely by providing medication to be self-administered.[24]

---

20. Ibid., 814–16.
21. Ibid., 818.
22. *Quill v. Vacco,* 80 F. 3rd 716 (2nd Cir. 1996).
23. Ibid., 718
24. Ibid., 718–19.

After losing in District Court, the three physicians appealed to the Second Circuit Court of Appeals. Circuit Judge Miner quoted approvingly the appeal for actions from his court as argued by Dr. Quill:

> The removal of a life support system that directly results in the patient's death requires the direct involvement by the doctor as well as other medical personnel. When such patients are mentally competent they are consciously choosing death as preferable to life under circumstances that they are forced to live. Their doctors do a careful clinical assessment, including a full exploration of the patient's prognosis, mental competence to make such decisions, and the treatment alternative to stopping treatment. It is legally and ethically permitted for physicians to actively assist patients to die who are dependent on life-sustaining treatments.... Unfortunately, some dying patients who are in agony that can no longer be relieved, yet are not dependent on life-sustaining treatment, have no such options under current legal restrictions. It seems unfair, discriminating, and inhumane to deprive some dying patients of such vital choices because of arbitrary elements of their condition which determines whether they are on life-sustaining treatment that can be stopped.[25]

Notice that Quill is portraying the physician as a causal agent in the death of a patient who dies after refusing life-sustaining treatment: the cessation of life support *results* in death. Based also on this consequentialist argument, the patient is depicted as one who *chooses* death, and does so in preference to continued life in the circumstances. In this classical utilitarian mode of reasoning, the rightness and wrongness of actions are judged by their consequences, and, as well, the intentions of actions are judged by what the action foreseeably brings about. Banning PAS is unfair because what the patient is requesting of the physician is no different ethically from requesting a physician to cease life-sustaining treatment that will result in death.

That Miner accepted Quill's argument is evident in the following passage:

---

25. Ibid., 721.

Moreover, the writing of a prescription to hasten death after consultation with a patient, involves a far less active role for the physician than is required in bringing about death through asphyxiation, starvation, and/or dehydration. Withdrawal of life support requires physicians or those acting at their direction physically to remove equipment and, often, to administer palliative drugs which may themselves contribute to death. The ending of life by these means is nothing more or less than assisted suicide. It simply cannot be said that those mentally competent, terminally ill patients who seek to hasten death but whose treatment does not include life support are treated equally.[26]

In this passage, Miner, like Quill, ascribed a causal role to the physician in the death of patients that follows after life-sustaining treatment has been refused or after palliative care using drug dosages that compromise life. Indeed, for Miner, these acts are acts of assisted suicide. In both cases, the result is death. By prohibiting PAS while permitting other medical practices that bring about death, New York is treating patients unequally, in violation of the requirement of laws that provide equal protection for everyone under their jurisdiction, as stated in the Fourteenth Amendment.

To make the case for reversing the decision of the Second Circuit Court of Appeals, Rehnquist, writing for the Supreme Court, expressly disputed the lower court's line of argumentation as quoted and interpreted above:

On their faces, neither the assisted suicide ban nor the law permitting patients to refuse medical treatment treats anyone differently from anyone else or draws any distinctions between persons. *Everyone* regardless of physical conditions, is entitled, if competent, to refuse unwanted lifesaving medical treatment; *no one* is permitted to assist a suicide. Generally laws that apply evenhandedly to all unquestionably comply with equal protection.... This Court disagrees with the Second Circuit's submission that ending or refusing lifesaving medical treatment "is nothing more or less than assisted suicide." The distinction between letting a patient die and making that patient die is important, logical, rational, and

---

26. Ibid., 729.

well established. It comports with fundamental legal principles of causation ... and intent ... and has been widely recognized and endorsed in the medical profession, the state courts, and the overwhelming majority of state legislatures which, like New York's, have permitted the former while prohibiting the latter. ... Logic and contemporary practice support New York's judgement that the two acts are different, and New York may therefore, consistent with the Constitution, treat them differently.[27]

Rehnquist then proceeded to fill out the arguments that the law has treated, and continues to treat, causation and intent very differently from the way in which Judge Miner and Dr. Quill depicted them.

Legal Principle of Causation. Contrasting starkly with Miner's portrayal of causation when a patient refuses life-sustaining medical interventions, courts, cited by Rehnquist, have depicted such a patient as dying "from an underlying" fatal disease or pathology; but a patient that "ingests lethal medications prescribed by a physician ... [as] killed by that medication."[28] Rehnquist also quoted the American Medical Association, Council on Ethical and Judicial Affairs, to the same effect. Unlike Reinhardt, Rehnquist respects and approves of their argument and their position.

Legal Principle of Intent. Physicians who comply with requests either to withdraw or not to begin life-sustaining treatment purposefully intend, or may so intend, only to respect the wishes of such patients and at the same time discontinue interventions deemed to be useless, futile, or degrading to patients who no longer stand to benefit from them.[29] The same holds in instances in which drugs that relieve pain may have the effect of hastening death: the physicians intend, or may intend, only to ease pain. Those physicians, however, who assist a suicide:

> "must necessarily and indubitably, intend primarily that the patient be dead." [Reference omitted] Similarly, a patient who commits suicide with a doctor's aid necessarily has the specific

---

27. *Vacco v. Quill*, 117 S.Ct. 2293 (1997), 2297–98.
28. Ibid., 2298.
29. Ibid.

intent to end his or her own life, while a patient who refuses or discontinues treatment might not.[30]

Once more, Rehnquist followed this with quotations from court decisions to the same effect.

Rehnquist then further documented how the law has interpreted, and continues to interpret, intent: "The law has long used actors' intent or purpose to distinguish between two acts that may have the same result."[31] This occurs in the common law regarding homicide when it "distinguishes...between a person who knows that another person will be killed as the result of his conduct and a person who acts with the specific purpose of taking another's life."[32] Formulating this in the very way typical of the "Rule of Double Effect," Rehnquist observed that "the law distinguishes actions taken 'because of' a given end from actions taken 'in spite of' their unintended but foreseen consequences."[33] At this point, Rehnquist called attention to the use of the Rule of Double Effect as an important mode of reasoning within law, the very rule that Judge Reinhardt was asking both judges and physicians to abandon in favor of a purely consequentialist mode of reasoning. For Reinhardt, what actors intend is discovered by what results from their actions. The reader should know that Rehnquist's arguments against Miner's opinions are also explicitly intended as a refutation of Reinhardt on this same matter of distinguishing PAS from actions intended only to relieve pain and that stop, or never start, life-sustaining treatment, because it is burdensome and of little or no benefit.

These latter actions might have the unintended result, even if foreseen, of hastening a patient's death, but they are nevertheless distinguishable in this intent from the intent of PAS, that of purposefully ending the patient's life with means known to be lethal. Of course, Rehnquist is not giving philosophical arguments for the Rule of Double Effect. Rather, he is appropriately enough indicating that it has had, and continues to have, a significant role in making legal decisions. This mode of arguing is, as I say, appropriate since it is in the context of deciding the constitutionality of a law, and law and facts are the acknowledged bases for such decisions.

---

30. Ibid., 2299.
31. Ibid.
32. Ibid.
33. Ibid.

There are also more nuanced arguments that lend support to Reinhardt and Miner by attacking the Rule of Double Effect and concluding that PAS, and what Rehnquist calls "letting die," are to be equated. These arguments will need to be spelled out and plausibly criticized before Rehnquist's position can be credibly defended. These matters, including a clarification of the terminology being used, such as the Rule of Double Effect, will be discussed below and in the final chapter.

What Rehnquist clearly does demonstrate is that the law and the medical profession, in the past and present, distinguish intended from unintended consequences, exhibiting in their deliberations and policies a mode of reasoning that is not, as in Mill, purely consequentialist. Therefore, the "right to refuse life-sustaining treatment" is not to be equated with the "right to hasten death."

Rehnquist also rejected Miner's consequentialist analysis in another important respect. Miner had referred to the Supreme Court's decision in the matter of *Cruzan* to bolster his opinion.[34] Rehnquist rejected Miner's interpretation of *Cruzan*:

> our assumption of a right to refuse treatment was grounded not, as the Court of Appeals supposed, on the proposition that patients have a general and abstract "right to hasten death," [Reference omitted] but on well established, traditional rights to bodily integrity and freedom from unwanted touching. [Reference omitted] In fact, we observed that "the majority of States in this country have laws imposing criminal penalties on one who assists another to commit suicide." [Reference omitted] *Cruzan*, therefore, provides no support for the notion that refusing life-sustaining medical treatment is "nothing more or less than suicide."[35]

On the basis of all the arguments Rehnquist has offered, he concluded, in summary, that the claim that "the distinction between refusing lifesaving medical treatment and assisted suicide is arbitrary and irrational, is mistaken."[36] So both "logic" and "contemporary practice" support New York's judgment that the two acts differ, and it is, therefore, consistent with the Constitution to

---

34. *Cruzan v. Director, Mo. Dept. of Health*, 497 U.S. 261 (1990).
35. *Vacco v. Quill*, 2301.
36. Ibid.

treat them differently. What New York law is doing, by permitting everyone to refuse medical treatment they do not wish and, at the same time, prohibiting anyone from assisting in a suicide, "follows a longstanding and rational distinction."[37]

We know that the Supreme Court also reversed the decision of the *en banc* Ninth Circuit Court of Appeals as articulated by Judge Reinhardt for the majority. Specifically the holding was that "Washington's prohibition against 'caus[ing]' or 'aid[ing]' a suicide does not violate the 'Due Process Clause' of the Fourteenth Amendment."[38] What the Due Process clause provides is more than a fair process; it provides "heightened protection against government interference with certain fundamental rights and liberty interests."[39] Among the rights protected is that of refusing "unwanted lifesaving medical treatment."[40] Strictly speaking, Rehnquist considered this particular liberty interest one that "may be inferred from our prior decisions."[41]

The holding may be described in still another way. Rehnquist noted that what the Washington law forbids is "aid[ing] another person to attempt suicide."[42] The question, then, to be decided is whether the "liberty" that the Due Process clause protects, "includes a right to commit suicide which itself includes a right to assistance in doing so."[43] The Supreme Court's answer to that question was: there is no such right; there is no such constitutionally protected liberty.

We can observe that this specification of the right asserted by the Ninth Circuit and rejected by the Supreme Court reflects the ac-

---

37. Ibid., 2302.
38. *Washington v. Glucksberg*, 117 S.Ct. 2258 (1997), 2259. On page 2275, the Court's holding is described as follows: "We therefore hold that Wash. Rev. Code 9A.36.060(1)(1994) does not violate the Fourteenth Amendment, either on its face or 'as applied to competent, terminally ill adults who wish to hasten their deaths by obtaining medication prescribed by their doctors.' " For an explanation of the technical concepts "on its face" and "as applied," see James Bopp, Jr., and Richard E. Coleson, "Three Strikes: Is an Assisted Suicide Right Out?" *Issues in Law and Medicine* 15, no. 1 (Summer 1999): 3–86 (see pages 37–52).
39. *Washington v. Glucksberg*, 2258.
40. Ibid., 2259.
41. Ibid., 2269. In *Cruzan*, the Supreme Court allowed Missouri to retain a law that permitted patients, under specified conditions, to discontinue the medical administration of nutrition and hydration. (See Rehnquist's discussion of this case on pages 2269–70.)
42. Ibid., 2269.
43. Ibid.

ceptance of the distinctions between refusing unwanted lifesaving medical treatment and requesting aid to commit suicide. Rehnquist did not accept the expression "hastening death," for it is the expression that conveys Reinhardt's collapse of the distinction between refusing unwanted lifesaving medical treatment and requesting aid to commit suicide. Furthermore, an expression such as "hastening death" is too broad and ambiguous, and in these ways is not in keeping with an important feature of what Rehnquist calls "substantive due process analysis" requiring as it has in past cases, "a 'careful description' of the asserted fundamental liberty interest."[44] Here again, the Supreme Court's analysis can take the form it does only because it is honoring the distinction between acts of refusing treatment, or palliative care, that may in some instances "hasten death" and acts that "hasten death" by known, lethal means.

The conflict between the position taken by Reinhardt and Miner, and that taken by Rehnquist and the entire Supreme Court, is not being directly engaged, not at least at the level of a philosophical debate over differing modes of moral argumentation with differing outcomes. Reinhardt and Miner are employing a particular, purely consequentialist mode of moral reasoning and mounting an argument for claiming that the distinction between refusing life-sustaining treatment and requesting assistance to commit suicide is arbitrary, irrational, or, in effect, incorrect. In turn, Rehnquist is rejecting these claims, not by fashioning his own philosophical argument against them, but by citing sources that make use of an alternative mode of moral reasoning. He found alternative modes of moral reasoning in court decisions, in common law, in legislation, and in ethical codes and practices of the medical profession. If PAS is ever to be sanctioned as a constitutionally protected liberty interest, it will have to develop much wider and deeper acceptance, ethically and legally, than it presently has. As Rehnquist noted in a description of his method of substantive-due-process analysis,

> The Due Process Clause protects those fundamental rights and liberties which are objectively, "deeply rooted in this nation's history and tradition, . . . " so rooted in the traditions and conscience of our people as to be ranked fundamental . . . " and

---

44. Ibid., 2268.

implicit in the concept of ordered liberty," such that, "neither liberty nor justice would exist if they were sacrificed."[45]

In asserting this, Rehnquist was quoting from past Supreme Court decisions.

Reinhardt and Miner clearly are not persuaded by these appeals to legal precedent, however appropriate in the context of deliberations over constitutional law. From a philosophical point of view, these are appeals to authority, not in themselves valid arguments for the point of view taken in these courts. They are well aware of these previous court decisions, but they reject their applicability to the decision over PAS. They do so on explicitly philosophical grounds, their own version of traditions based on Mill. Appeals to alternative traditions will not, by themselves, provide a rationale for abandoning their philosophical preferences. By calling attention to this conflict and the impasse created by it, I begin to address one of the problems dividing courts and judges who make decisions as members of a particular court. There are Millian and non-Millian traditions behind some of these divisions within courts as well as among them.

Because the particular version of Mill appearing in the courts is quite at odds with a longstanding consensus that originates in and persists beyond the Natural Rights Synthesis mentioned above, it is important to discover at least two things: the plausibility of this particular version of Mill; the possibility of forging a new consensus that is compatible with the earlier synthesis but attends to certain elements in Mill, neglected by American jurists, Reinhardt and Miner among them. It is important also to provide a justification for forging a new consensus, one that would at the same time provide a philosophical, ethical defense of the Supreme Court's legal and factual objections to PAS.

I begin these tasks in this chapter by examining philosophically nuanced arguments that would support Reinhardt and Miner's collapse of the distinction between refusing life-sustaining treatment and requesting aid in committing suicide. I conclude the chapter by taking issue with these arguments and, in doing so, begin to build a case for the traditions and for the current legal and ethical frame-

---

45. Ibid.

work in which PAS is regarded as legally and morally unjustified. But first, the terminology I will use needs to be clarified.

CRITICAL CONCEPTUAL ISSUES

Comfort-only care. This is the care that is to be distinguished from PAS. By comfort-only care, I mean to convey that the care being given a patient is aimed at the relief of pain and suffering. The resort to comfort-only care occurs when curative efforts are no longer regarded as efficacious. Whether all other life-sustaining interventions are to be refused, whether withheld or withdrawn, becomes a matter of evaluating how burdensome they are, relative to what benefits they may have. These decisions with respect to life-sustaining treatment not only have comfort in view; they may also seek to prolong life even while the patient is dying of a terminal disease, in order to accomplish certain purposes, such as taking leave of loved ones or finishing some project, given, of course, that a patient's condition allows for whatever energy and communicative abilities are necessary for such purposes. But pain relief can hasten death, and the refusal of life-sustaining modalities, such as a respirator, can quickly end life. Such examples raise the question of whether decisions of comfort-only care that clearly hasten death are in any way significantly different from decisions to request PAS, or even euthanasia, when curative efforts have been justifiably abandoned and the focus is on ending pain and suffering.

Suicide is the voluntary and intentional killing of oneself.[46] The term "voluntary" is essential to attributing the act that ends life to the agent whose life it is. The term "intentional" is used to contrast suicide as an act from an act that would be properly deemed to be accidental, as in the case of a gun assumed to be unloaded that discharges and kills the one who pressed the trigger. This terminology does not exclude the possibility that some or all acts of ending one's life may be done in a psychological state of depression such that, from a psychological point of view, the act is not rationally or totally "voluntary" in every sense of the word, and not rationally or totally "intentional" in every sense of that word.

---

46. With respect to defining "suicide" and "PAS," I am guided by Robert D. Orr, "The Physician-Assisted Suicide: Is It Ever Justified?" in *Suicide: A Christian Response*, ed. T. J. Demy and G. P. Stewart (Grand Rapids, Mich.: Kregel, 1998), chap. 4.

Physician-assisted suicide (PAS) occurs when a physician, knowing that the patient's intention is to commit suicide, provides the means used to carry it out, means such as information, prescriptions, or a "suicide machine."

Euthanasia, in its original meaning, referred to a "good death." It has come to mean "mercy killing." A mercy killing takes place when someone motivated by compassion intentionally and actively kills someone to end that individual's suffering. *Voluntary euthanasia* is carried out at the request of the individual whose life is ended; *involuntary euthanasia* is carried out without the request or consent of the individual whose life is ended; *nonvoluntary euthanasia* is carried out on incompetent individuals.

Discussions of PAS and euthanasia usually take up the distinction between *active* and *passive* euthanasia. The term "active euthanasia" is actually just another way to describe what has been defined as "euthanasia" in the paragraph immediately above. I will use the term "euthanasia" to refer only to "active euthanasia." "Passive euthanasia" is used to describe situations in which life-sustaining treatments are withheld or withdrawn from a terminally ill patient, allowing the individual to die naturally. The expressions "letting die" and "allowing to die" have also been applied to these same circumstances. I employ "comfort-only care" to refer to these kinds of situations. Since "euthanasia" has come to be associated with "mercy killing," it can be confusing as a description of situations that include, for example, refusing an experimental treatment that promises to prolong life but that could very likely also cause the death of a patient. What is being refused is high-risk intervention with its burdensome side effects in order to pursue other activities free of such risks and burdens. Comfort-only care appropriately depicts such situations. The terms "passive," "letting," and "allowing" are also less than satisfactory ways to describe how a physician is expected to relate to a patient who is dying. Patients who are dying need care, or assistance for obtaining care, such as nursing care at home, from the physicians who have judged that they are indeed beyond a cure. Comfort-only care is a clearer way to refer to these practices in medicine, since relief of pain and suffering is regarded as an obligation of physicians irrespective of what other medical interventions may or may not be involved when such an obligation exists toward a given patient.

Allowing to die or *letting die* are often considered to be morally different from killing. But correctly labeling an act as "allowing to die" does not tell us whether the act is morally justified. If, for example, an individual whose life could have been saved in an emergency room is knowingly and deliberately allowed to die, such inaction would be morally akin to an unjustified killing, given the moral and legal obligations to treat in such circumstances. (In this instance I am assuming that the time, resources, and medical personnel are all sufficient to save that individual's life.) At the same time, killing in defense of a life is generally accepted as morally and legally justified. A physician who had to use such force to defend herself against a patient turned violent that the patient died from the struggle may be said to have killed that patient, but justifiably, albeit tragically, under those circumstances. Resorting to comfort-only care also may sometimes be morally akin to killing if, for example, it is knowingly done for a patient who is judged to be curable by conventionally accepted medical means, who is not properly informed of that fact, or for whom no efforts to seek consent for treatment have been made.

Therefore, the question to which we now attend, the question of whether there is a moral difference between comfort-only care and PAS, is more precisely a question of whether comfort-only care can sometimes be morally justified whereas PAS never can be. As we will see, that discussion will require attention to euthanasia as well as PAS.

EQUATING SOME INSTANCES OF PAS WITH COMFORT-ONLY CARE

In the fourth edition of their text in bioethics, Tom Beauchamp and James Childress have argued in favor of PAS as a public policy and argued as well on behalf of the moral acceptability of PAS and euthanasia under exceptional and highly circumscribed circumstances.[47] A critical element in drawing these conclusions is to argue:

> If competent patients have a legal and moral right to refuse treatment that involves health professionals in implementing their decision and bringing about their deaths, we have a

47. Tom Beauchamp and James F. Childress, *Principles of Biomedical Ethics*, 4th ed. (New York: Oxford University Press, 1994).

reason to suppose they have a similar right to request the assistance of willing physicians to help them control the conditions under which they die. Assuming that omission of treatment is justified by the principles of respect for autonomy and nonmaleficence, cannot the same form of justification be extended to physicians prescribing barbiturates needed by seriously ill patients, and possibly to physician-administered lethal injections?[48]

Beauchamp and Childress note that this argument points to an apparent inconsistency: patients have a right based on their autonomy, in grim circumstances, to refuse treatment so as to bring about their deaths, but they are denied such a right, in equally grim circumstances, to arrange for their death by mutual agreement between themselves and their physicians. The authors believe that the need to exercise the right to have one's life ended with the help of a physician involves only a small percentage of patients because of the great strides in pain management, improved environments for patients, and the existence of hospice to care for the dying. But this does not suffice for all conditions in which patients find themselves, and Beauchamp and Childress add,

> ... in any event there are significant questions about autonomy rights for patients. If a right exists to stop a machine that sustains life, through an arrangement involving mutual agreement with a physician, why is there not the same right to stop the machine that *is* one's life by an arrangement with a physician?[49]

It is important to note that Beauchamp and Childress are not simply equating every act of refusing treatment with acts that are intended to end life. A patient may choose to discontinue a treatment that is futile to prevent death. In an example they provide, Beauchamp and Childress describe a situation in which an individual will live for one month more with or without continuing dialysis. When the patient in this case elects to stop dialysis treatments in order to be at home with loved ones, free of the machine and the

---

48. Ibid., 226.
49. Ibid., 224.

hospital, there is no suicidal intent as some have argued.[50] Suicide is the wrong category to apply and so, then, is PAS because death will result, with or without treatment, from untreatable conditions that are not arranged by the patient for the purpose of ending life: "This is what we might call a 'pure' refusal case that lacks all suicidal intent."[51]

But refusals of treatment "are instances of suicide whenever the agent specifically arranges the conditions to bring about death."[52] Since, in the view of Beauchamp and Childress, these refusals are generally morally and legally accepted under certain "grim" circumstances, there is no justifiable reason to ban PAS and even voluntary euthanasia under similarly "grim" circumstances. The autonomy of patients should be honored in both ways of choosing to die.

Under the Rule of Double Effect (hereafter RDE), refusals of treatment that are, or should be, morally accepted and legally recognized are never instances of suicide or anything morally equivalent. Refusals of treatment that knowingly result in death are not viewed as acts of suicide. In cases in which patients are terminally ill, for example, if physicians provide pain relief that has a substantial probability of shortening life, it is not considered PAS, and, unlike PAS, it is morally justifiable. In these same circumstances, providing a lethal injection (euthanasia) to end pain is regarded as wrongfully killing the patient, and the patient is wrongfully requesting such actions. What is morally justifiable is the provision of medication with the intention of relieving pain, *without in any way intending to hasten death*. If no intention of ending life with a known lethal effect exists in such a case, this act is morally justified because it does not directly and intentionally harm (kill) an innocent individual.

Beauchamp and Childress find fault with a key element in the RDE: "Adherents of the RDE need an account of intentional actions and intended effects of action (intentionally causing or allowing) that properly distinguishes them from nonintentional actions and unintended effects (foreseeably causing or allowing)."[53] This the

---

50. Ibid. Beauchamp and Childress give as an example of falsely assuming suicidal intent in all cases of refusing treatment necessary to prolong life, Dan Brock, "Death and Dying," in *Medical Ethics*, ed. Robert M. Veatch (Boston: Jones and Bartlett Publishers, 1989).
51. Beauchamp and Childress, *Principles of Biomedical Ethics*, 224.
52. Ibid.
53. Ibid. See pages 206–11 for their full description and critique of RDE and their footnote 41 for further discussions and viewpoints with respect to the uses of RDE.

RDE cannot provide. Beauchamp and Childress begin their reasons for this claim by calling attention to a view that is widely shared in an otherwise controversial literature on intention: intentional actions are characterized by an agent's plan, one that contains some representation of the means and ends being proposed. For an action to be deemed intentional, it has to be in accord with the agent's conception of how it was planned to be performed. Using "a model of intentionality based on what is *willed* rather than what is *wanted*," Beauchamp and Childress assert that "intentional actions and intentional effects include any action and any effect willed in accordance with a plan, including tolerated as well as wanted effects."[54]

Given this conception of intention, there is no viable distinction between what is intended and what is only foreseeable:

> Thus a person who knowingly and voluntarily acts to bring about an effect brings about that effect intentionally. The effect is intended, although the person did not desire it, did not will it for its own sake, or did not intend it as the goal of the action.[55]

This way of understanding intentional actions means that physicians who have pain relief as their goal, and whose interventions for that purpose also hasten death, have, at the same time, intentionally served as a causal agent in the deaths of such patients. If killing someone is described as causing someone's death, then one can view these deaths as examples of physicians killing patients. Legally they are not described in this way, nor do Beauchamp and Childress advocate that they be described in this way. Rather what they advocate is that hastening death by means of pain relief or refusal of life-sustaining treatment in the circumstances now generally sanctioned morally and legally should be recognized as no different morally from hastening death by PAS or euthanasia: all of these actions are morally the same—they cause the death of patients in very dire circumstances and they arrange their deaths through mutually agreed upon procedures. It should be noted that Beauchamp and Childress advocate the legalization of PAS, and though they favor euthanasia, they do not advocate legalizing it at the present time.

---

54. Ibid., 209.
55. Ibid.

Beauchamp and Childress have not resorted to the simpler arguments of some consequentialists, such as Reinhardt and Miner, that the practices they equate are morally indistinguishable because they both have the same effect, namely, that the patient's life is foreshortened. They have retained the very important concept of intention, the importance of which Rehnquist amply illustrated as indicated earlier. As Rehnquist observed in *Vacco v. Quill,*

> The law has long used actors' intent or purpose to distinguish between two acts that may have the same result.... ("[T]he ...common law of homicide often distinguishes... between a person who knows that another person will be killed as a result of his conduct and a person who acts with the specific purpose of taking another's life")... (distinctions based on intent are "universal and persistent in mature systems of law"). [All references have been omitted].[56]

Rehnquist concluded this paragraph with the language and reasoning of the RDE as embedded in law: "...the law distinguishes actions taken 'because of' a given end from actions taken 'in spite of' their unintended but foreseen consequences."[57] He then found that this same mode of reasoning, in law and by the medical profession, compelled the Supreme Court to reject the claim of the Second Circuit Court of Appeals that ending or refusing life-sustaining treatment "is nothing more or less than assisted suicide."[58]

But if Beauchamp and Childress are right about how the RDE should be interpreted, a simple appeal to it would not serve to reverse the decision of the Second Circuit Court of Appeals; nor would such an appeal serve as a critical element in reversing the decision of the Ninth Circuit Court of Appeals. Beauchamp and Childress have provided a much stronger argument than that of Reinhardt and Miner for justifying PAS when it is requested in circumstances that would also justify comfort-only treatment, but in which a patient and physician agree that PAS is the more humane or dignified way to end one's life.

Clearly, jurists would not be persuaded by Rehnquist's reasoning found in law, and we know some are not, if they rejected the

---

56. *Vacco v. Quill,* 2299.
57. Ibid.
58. *Quill v. Vacco,* 729.

RDE for the reasons offered by Beauchamp and Childress. But have Beauchamp and Childress defined intent and described causation in such a way that Rehnquist's reasoning as quoted above has to be rejected? I think not.

MORAL DIFFERENCES BETWEEN PAS AND COMFORT-ONLY CARE

To begin with, I find that Beauchamp and Childress have described intent and causation in a plausible way. I accept their conclusions that "intentional actions and intentional effects include any action and any effect willed in accordance with the plan, including toler- ated as well as wanted effects."[59] This means that what Rehnquist calls "foreseen consequences," as does the RDE, are to be viewed as intended, and the physician as the agent causing them, and so as the agent who shortens life in the instances in which that is the effect foreseen. What I wish to show is that one can accept their account of intent and this aspect of causal responsibility noted above and still affirm the moral differences identified by applying the RDE to instances of PAS, euthanasia, and comfort-only treatment. At the same time, I do not regard the RDE, as usually understood, as ad- equate to argue the case against PAS and euthanasia, for reasons that will become evident as my discussion proceeds.

Beauchamp and Childress do not dismiss every aspect of the RDE. They employ one of its "rules" in deciding what actions are morally justifiable. I refer to the principle of "proportionality" that would justifiably allow a harmful effect "only if a proportionately weighty good will probably be brought about.[60] In other words, one weighs the relation between burdens and benefits to help determine whether an act is morally justified. I want to begin my argument on this very point but describe this consideration in a somewhat different way.

The late eminent twentieth-century moral philosopher W. D. Ross observed that most actions are morally complex.[61] They are morally complex in the sense that they have more than one right- or wrong-making characteristic. One example would be an act that

---

59. Beauchamp and Childress, *Principles of Biomedical Ethics*, 209.
60. Ibid., 210–11.
61. W. D. Ross, *The Right and the Good* (Oxford: Oxford University Press, 1930), chap. 2.

is done for the sake of saving an accident victim, which act is at the same time an act that breaks a promise to meet a friend for dinner at a particular time. Instead of analyzing this as a case in which to apply the RDE, which would be applicable, Ross speaks of saving a life as the most right act in the circumstances. The act in question is right insofar as it is an act of saving a life but wrong insofar as it is an act of breaking a promise. To claim that saving a life is the most right thing to do and, as Ross would also claim, one's actual duty in the circumstances, is to consider saving a life as having more moral weight than keeping the particular promise in question. If, however, breaking a promise would result in the death of the one to whom the promise was made, Ross would view this as the most right action relative to saving someone else's life for two reasons: (1) keeping the promise satisfies two right-making characteristics; (2) nonmaleficence, refraining from harm, is generally more stringent (weighty) than beneficence, doing something good for another. For Ross, the rightness of acts depends upon what kinds of actions they are. Thus, refraining from harming others is right insofar as it is the refraining from inflicting harm. This is a morally significant way to relate to other persons. Another morally significant relation is one individuals have to themselves. Ross identifies duties of self-improvement, those of increasing in virtue or intelligence. In the analysis that follows, I will be seeking to identify morally significant relations that make up right- or wrong-making characteristics of actions. This will identify aspects of comfort-only care, PAS, and euthanasia not noticed or attended to by Beauchamp and Childress.

Let us begin with the example of increasing pain relief near the end of life to a degree that knowingly has a high probability of hastening death. Beauchamp and Childress would claim that engaging in this practice at the request of the terminally ill patient is an act that intends not only to relieve pain but also to end life. If this intentional hastening of death is morally acceptable, it should be equally morally acceptable to hasten death by providing a lethal dose of medication (PAS) or a lethal injection (euthanasia) at the request of a patient who requests it for relief of pain that would otherwise require massive, life-compromising dosages to relieve. Indeed, why not end the pain even more quickly, if that is agreeable to the physician and patient? At first blush these acts appear to share the same moral characteristics: the right-making characteristic of relieving pain and the wrong-making characteristic of ending a life.

But there are other morally significant aspects of these acts to consider. When physicians assist in a suicide or engage in euthanasia, they introduce into the physician/patient relation a lethal agent. Employing an agent known to be lethal relates the physician to the patient in one of the ways that someone who commits a premeditated murder relates to the one who is killed, namely, as one who fatally injures them with lethal means. The restraint against using means incompatible with the life of another human being has to be overcome. This directly undermines the usual inhibitions against killing that generally govern in human relations. In using an agent that relieves pain in dosages that are not known to be lethal until a dose becomes the final one, there is still an interaction with the patient as one who continues to live. Respect for the life of the patient persists, and in some cases, pain relief even successfully prolongs life and eases pain. In any event, when the patient dies in comfort-only care, it results from the interaction between the condition of the patient and the intervention, not from the intervention alone. Lethal means are the single cause of death in acts of PAS and euthanasia; the weakened condition of the patient is irrelevant to the cause of death. The one using medication to relieve pain is concerned about the condition of the patient as a living individual up to the moment of death. The inhibition against killing is no more adversely affected, if it is at all, than in undertaking high risk, emergency surgery to save a life, and failing. Furthermore, in the case of a terminally ill patient, you know that the death of the patient is not something you can prevent, only delay, by providing pain relief in measured amounts rather than amounts known to be immediately lethal. This is respect for life. This is refraining from killing unjustifiably as we usually understand it, that is, refraining from the use of means known to be lethal *in themselves,* or *as used,* for the purpose of ending someone's life.

Respect for life also entails the wish that the other individual live. There is no necessity to give up that wish when one is not engaging in acts using means that are known to kill. The physician remains willing to care for the patient; the patient remains willing to be cared for. Someone like Quill sees no value in these few extra days or even weeks, living in such dependence on the help of others. He is utterly opposed to laws that do not allow PAS for patients whose pain, in the end, can only be controlled by sedation. Respect for life should be reserved for a life that the patient would deem to be worth living. Beauchamp and Childress also stress what they consider to be the centrality of quality-of-life judgments.[62] They reject the proposal of the ethicist Paul Ramsey to limit judgments about when it is justifiable to refuse life-sustaining treatments to strictly medical indications.[63] For permanently unconscious patients, and that could include patients fully sedated in their last hours or days, they do not regard what they refer to as "mere biological life" to be a benefit. Maintenance of such a life could only be a benefit if the diagnosis or prognosis is wrong or a medical breakthrough occurs before the individual dies.

Ramsey opposes this shift, from assessing whether treatments are beneficial to patients to assessing whether patients' lives are beneficial to them. Beauchamp and Childress reject the basis of Ramsey's objection to this shift, namely, that it opens the door to involuntary euthanasia. But Ramsey has uncovered a critical element about treatment decisions. Once we begin to ground decisions that may result in hastening death or immediate death on an evaluation of the quality of anyone's life, we have introduced a mode of moral thinking that views some patients as having such a low quality of life that it is better for them to die than to receive comfort-only care. That is exactly one justification offered by Dutch physicians who violate the guidelines that permit voluntary euthanasia: they end the lives of some competent patients without their consent because these patients have such a low quality of life at the time and prospectively.[64] Ramsey's point has certainly proved plausible, possibly totally correct, though Beauchamp and Childress, as well as others, remain unpersuaded for reasons I will explore more fully in the concluding chapter. What occupies us now is that Beauchamp and Childress do not at this juncture give credence to a very important moral element that distinguishes comfort-only treatment from PAS and euthanasia. I refer to the manifestation of respect for life

---

62. Beauchamp and Childress, *Principles of Biomedical Ethics*, 215–19.
63. Ibid., 215–16.
64. See, for example, John Koewn, "Euthanasia in the Netherlands: Sliding Down the Slippery Slope?" *Notre Dame Journal of Law, Ethics and Public Policy* 9, no. 2 (1995), citing on p. 428 data showing that in 31 percent of a thousand cases of involuntary euthanasia, physicians gave "low quality of life" as their justification for such acts. See also Henk Jochemsen, "The Netherlands Experiment," in *Dignity and Dying*, ed. John F. Kilner, Arlene B. Miller, and Edmund D. Pellegrino (Grand Rapids, Mich.: Eerdmans, 1996). Both authors refer to a number of other published analyses of these same data and practices.

that takes place whenever physicians and patients regard human life as of *incalculable worth,* and therefore refuse to base their decision on any calculation of its worth. Hence, one reason for choosing sedation rather than PAS or euthanasia is that being sedated for pain relief is like living one's last days sleeping, and living this way does symbolize that the worth of one's life in that condition is not being questioned but respected.

There is another moral reason for choosing sedation and, more generally, comfort-only care rather than PAS or euthanasia. Comfort-only care allows one to sustain the quest to live a virtuous life, and even to gain in virtue, during one's very last days, weeks, months, or years on earth. With comfort-only care, you can witness to the incalculable worth of human life and the importance of discouraging others from resorting to suicide or euthanasia. By choosing comfort-only care rather than PAS or euthanasia, patients also help retain, in other patients and physicians, the inhibitions against using lethal means to end life directly. These inhibitions certainly have been weakened in Dutch physicians who do not even make the effort to obtain informed consent before deliberately ending the lives of competent patients. Judge Sopinka, writing for the Canadian Supreme Court, explicitly characterized an absolute ban on assisted suicide as an effort to prevent anyone tempted to commit suicide from doing so.[65] In this way Sopinka is portraying one thing he expects from the law, namely, an inhibitory effect on behavior that is destructive of human life.

Beauchamp and Childress might find some of these additional morally significant relations interesting, and may even agree that they merit discussion. However, they could argue that they too respect life and they favor safeguards against involuntary euthanasia as well as good faith efforts to offer alternatives to PAS and euthanasia. But in the last analysis, the individual who requests a quick painless death and the physician who complies should be free, by mutual agreement, to act accordingly. They do not view these actions as in any way morally unjustifiable. No one should or need be harmed by PAS or euthanasia under the conditions that justify comfort-only care. The decisions to resort to PAS or euthanasia involve respect for the autonomy of the agents. They do nothing that is inconsistent with virtue. Indeed, respect for autonomy is, for them,

---

65. *Rodriguez v. British Columbia,* 107 D.L.R. 4th 342 (1993).

a moral principle. Furthermore, Beauchamp and Childress take the view that, if an individual "desires death rather than life's more typical goods and projects, then causing that person's death at his or her autonomous request does not either harm or wrong the person (though it might still harm others—or society—by setting back their interests, which might be a reason against the practice)."[66] In their view, the wrong in killing is that the individuals killed are deprived of interests they might otherwise pursue and lose the very capacity to plan and choose a future in pursuit of their interests. But if an individual desires death, Beauchamp and Childress presume that they have no further interests they wish to pursue and so cannot be harmed by taking their lives or having them taken. One could say that for Beauchamp and Childress life has lost all of its worth, at least all worth that may be regarded as morally significant. Add to this account that individuals who see no worth in pursuing life plan to escape from suffering, and it is then the case that denying their plans is the harm that should be avoided. So, at least, Beauchamp and Childress contend.

Having identified to their satisfaction the elements that make killing wrong, Beauchamp and Childress return to the central concern discussed in this chapter when they conclude that

> those who believe it is sometimes morally acceptable to let people die but not to take active steps to help them die must therefore give a different account of the wrongfulness of killing persons than the one we have suggested. The burden of justification, then, seems to rest on those who would refuse assistance to those who wish to die, rather than on those who would help them.[67]

Beauchamp and Childress are certainly right that those who morally justify some instances of comfort-only care but no instances of PAS and euthanasia must give "a different account of the wrongfulness of killing" than the one they suggest. Indeed, that is precisely what we will find in the conflict between Rehnquist and Reinhardt—different accounts of the wrongfulness of killing. But in claiming that those who find PAS and euthanasia morally unjustifiable have the burden of proof, they are begging the question about whether

---

66. Beauchamp and Childress, *Principles of Biomedical Ethics*, 236.
67. Ibid.

comfort-only care differs morally from PAS and euthanasia. In the end, their failure to find a moral difference between comfort-only care and PAS and euthanasia rests on their particular claims as to what it is that makes killing wrong. They find nothing morally wrong about giving approval to a request for lethal means to end life from those who can find no purpose in continuing life. The request for comfort-only care, I will be arguing, if it is to be morally approved, should have as its purpose acting in a way that helps sustain the incalculable worth of human life for everyone, even in circumstances that would tempt some to think that life has lost all purpose. In taking up what is wrong about killing, it will become evident that the role they give to autonomy must be challenged. After all, there are good reasons why the law has never accepted the consent of the victim as a defense against the charge of wrongfully killing, that is, of murdering.

We turn now to consider further how Rehnquist and Reinhardt differ, especially on this question of the very basis for protecting life. It will be necessary to develop further, as I will, arguments against the views espoused by Beauchamp and Childress and discussed in this chapter, for their views are shared by some jurists, Reinhardt among them.

3

What Makes Killing Wrong

BY DESCRIBING AND ANALYZING the court decisions regarding PAS, we have seen the conflicting modes of moral reasoning and underlying premises that reflect differing moral and theological traditions. We noted also how the special version of Mill has the effect of changing the laws in ways that would suppress these other ways of thinking and the legal structures that embody them. In this chapter, we will see some further ways in which this would happen if PAS were to be constitutionally protected in accord with the *en banc* Ninth Circuit's decision, as articulated by Judge Reinhardt. Finally, a continuing discussion of what makes killing wrong when it is wrong will be a major concern in this chapter as we compare the reasoning of the Ninth Circuit with the reasoning of the Supreme Court, that is, the reasoning of these courts as expressed by Judge Reinhardt and Chief Justice Rehnquist respectively. This comparison will assist in the recovery of aspects of the legal tradition that have been suppressed in moral argumentation on the issue of assisted suicide and will also provide the foundation for forming a synthesis of traditions that protects the value of human life.

REINHARDT'S LIMITED PROTECTION OF HUMAN LIFE

Although Reinhardt, writing for the Ninth Circuit Court of Appeals, passionately defended a constitutional right to seek the assistance of a physician for the sake of committing suicide, he was well aware that the state does have an interest in preserving life and that this encompasses an interest in preventing suicide. Citing *Cruzan*, he made this point as follows:

As the court said in *Cruzan*, "we think that a State may properly decline to make judgments about the quality of life that a particular individual may enjoy, and simply assert an unqualified interest in the preservation of human life.... " [Reference omitted] Thus, the state may assert its interest in preserving life in all cases, including those of terminally ill, competent adults who wish to hasten their deaths."[1]

Indeed, he found it "distressing" that in the state of Washington during 1991, "suicide was the second leading cause of death after accidents for the age groups 15–19, 20–24, and 25–34, and one of the top five causes of death for age groups 35–44 and 45–54."[2] However, Reinhardt argues that the state's otherwise legitimate interest in preventing suicides is "considerably diminished" when individuals "are terminally ill, competent adults who wish to die."[3] A life ended prematurely is, for him, a "senseless" loss of life. For a terminally ill adult "ending life in the final stages of an incurable and painful degenerative disease, is only to avoid debilitating pain and a humiliating death,...[and] is not senseless, and death does not come too early."[4] And the state's interest in preventing death in such instances is not only "of comparatively little weight, but its insistence on frustrating their wishes seems cruel indeed."[5]

In these passages from Reinhardt's opinion, one can clearly discern two important elements found in the Millian tradition. In the first instance, Reinhardt, like Mill, clearly rejects the theological anthropology expressed by Hobbes by rejecting any assumption that individuals who are rational have a natural, continuous urge to preserve their own lives. Secondly, in the absence of such a natural, continuous proclivity to preserve one's own life, Reinhardt is asserting that a terminally ill person can sensibly calculate that life has so little pleasure or so much pain near its end that ending life becomes a rational act. This is unlike the conviction in Jewish and Christian sources that life's worth is beyond calculation. In fact, Reinhardt explicitly acknowledges "that judicial acceptance of physician-assisted suicide would cause many sincere persons with strong moral or reli-

---

1. *Compassion in Dying v. State of Washington*, 79 F. 3rd (9th Cir. 1996), 817.
2. Ibid., 820.
3. Ibid.
4. Ibid., 820–21.
5. Ibid., 821.

gious convictions great distress."[6] At that point, however, he noted that decisions to affirm a right to PAS should be accepted as valid judicial decisions no different from the judicial decisions already made to accommodate cases that invoke a double effect, as in comfort-only care. He observed also that what most distinguishes medical doctors who oppose PAS from those who favor its legalization is "a strong religious identification."[7] They also are admonished to abandon the doctrine of "double effect."

Although, therefore, Reinhardt was aware of his departure from the traditions currently representing a synthesis within American law, he was fully prepared to substitute his particular version of the Millian tradition. This he did knowingly. In a footnote to the work of Judge Richard Posner, Reinhardt took no issue with the argument that laws that ban assisted suicide (as they apply to the terminally ill) "violate Millsian [sic] principles and should, as a matter of policy, be repealed."[8] Reinhardt did take issue with Posner's view that the states should decide the laws regarding assisted suicide because of the moral values involved, and because a national rule would be premature. Reinhardt wanted to avoid protracted legal battles over patients who seek relief from more permissive states, and who may not obtain such relief in time to do any good. And, as we saw earlier, Reinhardt claimed that in this case the liberty interest is so important that it should be protected against states that would prohibit its exercise. In addition, while the state's interest in protecting life is very low, this important liberty interest is "at its height" for a competent adult patient who is terminally ill and wishes to die.[9]

Interestingly enough, Reinhardt gave liberty interests more weight than the right to life at the very outset. He cited approvingly a very early judicial expression of a Millian principle by Justice Brandeis in 1928:

> The makers of our Constitution undertook to secure conditions favorable to the pursuit of happiness.... They sought to protect Americans in their beliefs, their thoughts, their

---

6. Ibid., 824.
7. Ibid., 829.
8. Ibid., 833–34, footnote 124.
9. Ibid., 834. See also Ruth Russell, *Freedom to Die: Moral and Legal Aspects of Euthanasia* (New York: Human Sciences Press, 1975).

emotions and their sensations. They conferred, as against the government, the right to be let alone—the most comprehensive of rights, and the right most valued by civilized men.[10]

Note that rights are depicted as "conferred," not "natural," and the "right to be let alone" is "the right most valued." In Mill's essay "On Liberty" he regarded it as "progressive" to increase the sphere of life free from government coercion and required that societies not yet sufficiently educated or civilized be ruled nondemocratically until the people were ready for the increased liberties appropriate to democracies. This Millian thread in American law was observed and shaped earlier in 1890 in an article Brandeis wrote with Samuel D. Warren:

> That the individual shall have full protection in person and in property is a principle as old as the common law; but it has been found necessary from time to time to define anew the exact nature and extent of such protection.... Gradually the scope of these legal rights [to life, liberty, and property] broadened and now the right to life has come to mean the right to enjoy life,—the right to be let alone.[11]

Were these authors to share the theological anthropology espoused by Hobbes, they would not portray the natural inalienable right to life as "the right to be let alone" or "the right to enjoy life." For Hobbes, it was true, as it was for Mill, that human beings by nature seek pleasure and avoid pain for themselves, but for Hobbes, unlike Mill, human beings also seek to preserve their own lives. Reinhardt clearly presumed the Millian account of human nature in which he can regard it as "sensible" for individuals to calculate that their lives are not and will no longer be a source of happiness, and so would value more highly than continued life the freedom to avoid the pain, stress, or indignity of it.

Furthermore, when patients wish to have physicians aid them to end lives they no longer regard as a source of happiness, they are acting on a highly personal desire and set of beliefs. Like Mill, Rein-

---

10. Ibid., 800.
11. Samuel D. Warren and Louis D. Brandeis, "The Right to Privacy," *Harvard Law Review*, no. 4 (1890): 193. See also Nina Clark, *The Politics of Physician Assisted Suicide* (New York: Garland Publishing, 1997).

hardt asserts the existence of a sphere of sovereignty over one's own mind and body, a sphere that should be free from the interference of governments. Indeed, Reinhardt believes that the rationale for protecting a constitutional right to PAS is to be found in the Supreme Court's wording of its decision in *Casey*. Reinhardt cited what he sees as the relevant passage:

> These matters, involving the most intimate and personal choices a person may make in a lifetime, choices central to personal dignity and autonomy, are central to the liberty protected by the Fourteenth Amendment. At the heart of liberty is the right to define one's own concept of existence, of meaning, of the universe and of the mystery of human life. Belief about these matters could not define the attributes of personhood were they formed under the compulsion of the state.[12]

When the Supreme Court spoke of "these matters," it had reference to the "constitutional protection" the Court had previously afforded to personal choices as they relate to marriage, procreation, contraception, family relationships, child rearing, and education. To find a more direct link between choosing to end one's life as a personal choice and other previously protected personal choices, Reinhardt turned to the *Cruzan* decision.[13] Rehnquist, who wrote for the majority, was quoted by Reinhardt as saying that "the principle that a competent person has a constitutionally protected liberty interest in refusing unwanted medical treatment may be inferred from our prior decisions."[14] Since Reinhardt regards refusal of life-sustaining treatment as no different ethically or constitutionally from PAS, he claimed that a constitutionally recognized "right to die," based on *Casey* and *Cruzan,* already exists.[15]

Before elaborating further on Reinhardt's decision and its Millian presuppositions, I wish to document Rehnquist's reply to each of Reinhardt's arguments as presented so far.

---

12. *Compassion in Dying v. State of Washington* (1996), 813. See also Lewis Petrinovich, *Living and Dying Well* (New York: Plenum Press, 1996).
13. *Cruzan v. Director, Mo. Dept. of Health,* 497 U.S. 261(1990).
14. *Compassion in Dying v. State of Washington* (1996), 814, quoting *Cruzan* 497 U.S. at 278, 110 S.Ct. at 2851.
15. Ibid., 816 and 824.

REHNQUIST'S APPEAL TO RETAIN
THE CURRENT PROTECTIONS OF HUMAN LIFE

Life, the Right to Which Is Sacred, Natural, and Inalienable. As we have noted in the previous chapter, Rehnquist's method, for which there is ample precedent, in deciding due process cases, is to examine "our Nation's history, legal traditions, and practices."[16] What resulted from applying this method is that Rehnquist found that virtually every state and western democratic nation treats assisting in a suicide as a crime.[17] Rehnquist regarded these bans of assisted suicide as "longstanding expressions of the State's commitment to the protection and preservation of all human life."[18] Citing an earlier court, Rehnquist observed that the existence of such a "pattern of enacted laws" is "the primary and most reliable indication of [a national] consensus; and he adds the comment that "opposition to and condemnation of suicide—and, therefore, of assisting suicide— are consistent and enduring themes of our philosophical, legal, and cultural heritages."[19] Indeed, disapproval of both suicide and assisting suicide has persisted for over seven hundred years from the very origins of Anglo-American common-law tradition and even five centuries longer if one's reckoning includes England's adoption of the ecclesiastical prohibition on suicide.[20]

In what manner and on what basis was such opposition to suicide and assisting in it expressed? In the legislature of Rhode Island in 1647, for example, "self-murder" was described as "unnatural" and as in other early American colonies punished in accord with the common law of those times.[21] Common-law penalties began to be abolished in the eighteenth century. Zephaniah Swift, a legal scholar, later Chief Justice of Connecticut, writing in favor of abolishing all penalties against anyone committing suicide, nevertheless described suicide as "abhorrent to the feelings of mankind and that love of life which is implanted in the human heart."[22] Even when suicide was no longer regarded as a felony, the one who advised

---

16. *Washington v. Glucksberg,* 117 S.Ct. 2258 (1997), 2262.
17. Ibid., 2263. See footnote 8 for Rehnquist's sources, including Judge Beezer's dissent opposing Reinhardt's reasoning.
18. Ibid.
19. Ibid.
20. Ibid. Attend to footnote 9, as well as the text.
21. Ibid., 2264.
22. Ibid.

another to commit suicide, when the other actually killed himself as a result of this advice, was considered to be guilty of murder.

One might argue that if the person who is killed or kills himself consents to the aid or advice of another, the one who is giving aid or advice should not be treated as guilty of murder. But such is not the case. The principle in law is that "the consent of a homicide victim is wholly immaterial to the guilt of the person who cause[d] [his or her death]...."[23] The rationale for this can be found in twentieth-century sources cited by Rehnquist. In 1946 a Virginia court put it this way: "The right to life and to personal security is not only sacred in the estimation of the common law, but it is inalienable."[24] In 1980 the American Law Institute, in its Model Penal Code, prohibited "aiding" suicide and stimulated many states to enact explicit bans of assisted suicide:

> The Code's draftees observed that "the interests in the sanctity of life that are represented by the criminal homicide laws are threatened by one who expresses a willingness to participate in taking the life of another, even though the act may be accomplished with the consent, or at the request, of the suicide victim."[25]

It is not difficult to discern the "Puritan" and "Hobbesian" elements woven together in these characterizations of how and why the protection of life should include the prohibition of assisted suicide. Note that suicide is described as "unnatural" and "abhorrent to" the love of life implanted in the human heart, that is, human beings are depicted as naturally inclined to preserve their own lives, something both the Puritans and Hobbesian theological anthropologies affirmed. Furthermore, speaking of the "right to life" as "sacred" and inalienable weaves together the ideas of a natural inclination of divine origin with the Hobbesian view of this natural inclination as the basis for a "right that is inalienable." The expression "sanctity of life" continues in law to refer to the interest being protected by criminal homicide law, including as criminal homicide any aid given to a suicide victim who consented to or requested such aid.[26]

---

23. Ibid., 2265.
24. Ibid.
25. Ibid.
26. See, for example, *Bouvia v. Superior Court*, 225 Cal. Rptr. 297 (Cal. App. 2 Dist. 1986), 306. At this point, the court asserts that it is a crime to aid in a suicide,

Given these traditions within legislation and constitutional law, the version of Mill espoused by Reinhardt is in direct conflict with how these traditions view the right to life and its protection and implicitly in conflict with theological anthropologies reflected in the view taken by these traditions. Reinhardt thinks it makes sense to assist someone to commit suicide who is near death and no longer enjoys life. He does not presuppose a natural and persistent inclination toward self-preservation, nor a natural and inalienable right based on such an inclination, nor even a "sacredness" to the life of one who does not wish to live in a dying, suffering state. But the law, drawing on the traditions Reinhardt rejects, has not made exceptions to its prohibitions against assisting suicide for those who are near death. Rather, as Rehnquist observed, quoting legal sources,

> [t]he life of those to whom life ha[d] become a burden—of those who [were] hopelessly diseased or fatally wounded— nay, even the lives of criminals who were condemned to death [were] under the protection of law, equally as the lives of those who [were] in the full tide of life's enjoyment, and anxious to continue to live.[27]

Once again, the Puritan and Hobbesian natural rights traditions underlie and make sense of this legal practice. For the Puritans, the lives of individuals are equally worthy and of a worth beyond human calculations: as biblically portrayed, human beings are equally offspring of God and equally created in God's image.[28] For Hobbes, the right to life is inalienable for all human beings, and it would be irrational to try to relinquish that right. Such irrational behavior is to be prevented, not aided, so far as the state is concerned.

Considering the underlying premises that support the legal protection of human life, it comes as no surprise that Rehnquist would reaffirm as he did an "unqualified interest in the preservation of human life," and apply it to Washington law as he did to Missouri law in the quote from *Cruzan*.[29] This protection of individual

---

a law expressing the state's interest "in preserving and recognizing the sanctity of life," as stated in an earlier California Supreme Court decision, *In Re Joseph* (1983).

27. *Washington v. Glucksberg*, 2265.

28. See Genesis 1:27 and 31. Genesis, as most readers know, is a biblical book found in both the Hebrew and Christian scriptures.

29. *Washington v. Glucksberg*, 2272.

human life by banning assisted suicide is at the same time protection of the sanctity of life. For this he quoted again from the Model Penal Code of 1980 to the effect that the state's interests in the sanctity of life are "threatened" by anyone who would be willing to be a participant in taking another person's life, even if doing so is "with the consent, or at the request" of one who commits suicide.[30] Rehnquist regarded this interest as "symbolic and aspirational as well as practical," ideas he found well expressed by the New York State Task Force on Life and the Law:

> While suicide is no longer prohibited or penalized, the ban against assisted suicide and euthanasia shores up the notion of limits in human relationships. It reflects the gravity with which we view the decision to take one's own life or the life of another, and our reluctance to encourage or promote these decisions.[31]

Furthermore, this interest in protecting human life is unqualified in the sense that it is continuous and does not diminish in strength or "weight," for it does not depend, as Reinhardt alleged, "on the medical condition and the wishes of the person whose life is at stake."[32] After all, as the Supreme Court ruled in *Cruzan*, states "may properly decline to make judgments about the 'quality' of life that a particular individual may enjoy."[33] Washington State, therefore, has "properly" rejected Reinhardt's "sliding-scale approach and, through its assisted-suicide ban, insists that all persons' lives from beginning to end, are under the full protection of the law."[34]

In line with his support for protecting life, including that of those who may be distressed and/or near death, and in line with the aspirational aspect of the prohibition of assisted suicide, Rehnquist claimed that the state interest in preventing suicide is rationally related to its ban of assisted suicide. Rehnquist took cognizance of the considerable data that stress the high degree to which those who commit suicide had a major psychiatric illness at the time of death; some put the figure at 95 percent.[35] He took note also of

30. Ibid., 2272 and earlier at 2265.
31. Ibid., 2272.
32. Ibid.
33. Ibid.
34. Ibid.
35. Ibid.

the high degree to which suicidal, terminally ill patients respond well to treatment for depression and pain relief and are afterwards grateful to be alive; many who requested assisted suicide withdraw those requests after being treated for depression and pain.[36] Attention to these data underlie the traditions in law of presuming that human beings love life and seek to preserve their own lives, and that seeking to end one's life when terminally ill and close to death is not necessarily "sensible" or rational. Indeed, Rehnquist could have cited data and psychiatrists alleging that those who wish to commit suicide are always in need of treatment, often for clinical depression.[37] These data support, and these psychiatrists assume or espouse, a Hobbesian theological anthropology insofar as it depicts humans as naturally seeking to preserve their own lives.

When Rehnquist called attention to the fact that patients treated for pain often withdraw their requests for PAS, he could again cite further data and numerous individually dramatic cases.[38] The fact that the states of Washington and New York legally permit patients to choose comfort-only treatment was an important factor in achieving a unanimous decision in the Supreme Court to uphold the constitutionality of their laws. Justice O'Connor, in summarizing her concurring opinion, put great weight on palliative care as an alternative to PAS:

> In sum, there is no need to address the question whether suffering patients have a constitutionally cognizable interest in obtaining relief from the suffering that they may experience in the last days of their lives. There is no dispute that dying patients in Washington and New York can obtain palliative care, even when doing so would hasten their deaths. The difficulty in defining terminal illness and the risk that a dying patient's request for assistance in ending his or her life might not be

36. Ibid., 2273.

37. See, for example, Peter Sainsbury, "Community Psychiatry," in *A Handbook for the Study of Suicide,* ed. Seymour Perlin (New York: Oxford University Press, 1975), and J. H. Brown et al., "Is it Normal for Terminally Ill Patients to Desire Death?" *American Journal of Psychiatry* 143, no. 2 (February 1986): 208–11.

38. See, for example, Robert G. Twycross, "Where there is hope, there is life: a view from the hospice," in *Euthanasia Examined: Ethical, Clinical, and Legal Perspectives,* ed. John Keown (Cambridge: Cambridge University Press, 1995), 141–68. See also David Condiff, *Euthanasia Is Not the Answer: A Hospice Physician's View* (Clifton, N.J.: Humana Press, 1992).

truly voluntary justifies the prohibition on assisted suicide we uphold here.[39]

Justice Breyer, who concurred with the judgments expressed by O'Connor, departed from the Court's delineation of the "liberty interest" at stake: he preferred to call it a "right to die with dignity." Whatever the words used it could refer to the interests of "personal control over the manner of death, professional medical assistance, and the avoidance of unnecessary and severe physical suffering— combined."[40] But, in his view, "This Court does not need or now should decide whether or not such a right is fundamental."[41] That is true, for Breyer, because the claim to any right to PAS is compromised when severe pain can be avoided, and the laws before the Court do not force a dying person to experience that kind of pain. However, he underlined the importance of pain relief when he ended his opinion as follows:

> ...were state law to prevent the provision of palliative care, including the administration of drugs needed to avoid pain at the end of life—then the law's impact upon serious and otherwise unavoidable physical pain (accompanying death) would be more directly at issue. And as Justice O'Connor suggests, the Court might have to revisit its conclusions in these cases.[42]

As it turns out, then, no justice on the Supreme Court stood ready to accept Reinhardt's argument that it is cruel to reject some requests for PAS based on the state's interest in preserving life.[43] Nor did they accept his concluding indictment of those who would persist in the view that PAS should be legislatively prohibited as "compel[ling] those whose values differ from theirs to die painful, protracted, and agonizing deaths."[44] Certainly the Supreme Court did not regard the laws of Washington and New York states as vulnerable to Reinhardt's charge that legislatures and the will of the majority are imposing suffering on some patients.[45]

---

39. *Washington v. Glucksberg*, 2303. It should be noted that Justices Ginsberg and Breyer concurred with Justice O'Connor's opinion, although Breyer wrote a separate opinion. (See footnotes 40–42 for Breyer's reasons.)
40. Ibid., 2311.
41. Ibid.
42. Ibid., 2312.
43. *Compassion in Dying v. State of Washington*, 79 F. 3rd (9th Cir. 1996), 821.
44. Ibid., 839.
45. Some philosophers and physicians have argued that the waiting periods nec-

But Reinhardt and those who share his view are not convinced by the argument that permitting PAS is not necessary so long as sufficiently aggressive palliative care is legally permitted. As far as Reinhardt is concerned, the decision with respect to the time and manner of one's death is so personal and intimate that, as we observed earlier, it belongs to that sphere of privacy that Reinhardt regards as a decision that should remain free of government interference. And as we also observed earlier, Reinhardt maintained that the Supreme Court in *Cruzan* has already recognized such a right to determine the manner and timing of one's death, and in *Casey* has accepted as fundamental rights liberty interests that are personal and intimate. Rehnquist rejected Reinhardt's understanding of these decisions and the inferences he drew from them.

The *Cruzan* case considered whether Nancy Beth Cruzan had a constitutionally protected right such that the hospital would be required to withdraw life-sustaining treatment at her parents' request: she had been severely injured in an automobile accident and was diagnosed as being in a persistent vegetative state.[46] The Court examined: (1) the common law, in which it is a battery even to touch another person without that person's consent and without legal justification; and (2) the related rule generally requiring informed consent for medical treatment. "After reviewing a long line of relevant state cases, we concluded," said Rehnquist of the *Cruzan* case, "that the common law doctrine of informed consent is viewed as generally encompassing the right of a competent individual to refuse medical treatment."[47] On the basis of previous Supreme Court decisions on the same subject, the Court in *Cruzan* stated that "[t]he principle that a competent person has a constitutionally protected liberty interest in refusing unwanted medical treatment, may be inferred from our prior decisions."[48] For all of these reasons, the Court assumed that such a constitutionally protected liberty inter-

essary to assure correct diagnoses, reliable prognoses, and voluntariness before granting PAS are such that patients could die painlessly and as quickly from the withdrawal of nutrition and hydration under circumstances now regarded, incorrectly, as requiring PAS. For this argument, see Bernard Gert, Charles M. Culver, and K. Danner Clouser, "An Alternative to Physician-Assisted Suicide: A Conceptual and Moral Analysis," in *Physician-Assisted Suicide: Expanding the Debate*, ed. M. P. Battin, R. Rhodes, and A. Silver (New York: Routledge, 1998), 182–202.

46. *Washington v. Glucksberg*, 2269.
47. Ibid., 2270, quoting *Casey*.
48. Ibid., quoting *Cruzan*.

est, for purposes of the *Cruzan* case, would include a "right to refuse lifesaving hydration and nutrition."[49] Even so the Court took the view that "the Constitution permitted Missouri to require clear and convincing evidence of an incompetent patient's wishes concerning the withdrawal of life-sustaining treatment."[50]

Reinhardt had claimed that recognizing a liberty interest that includes the refusal of life-sustaining food and water "necessarily recognized a liberty interest in hastening one's own death."[51] To that, Rehnquist replied directly that:

> the right assumed in *Cruzan,* however, was not simply deduced from abstract concepts of personal autonomy.... The decision to commit suicide with the assistance of another may be just as personal and profound as the decision to refuse unwanted medical treatment but it has never enjoyed similar legal protection. Indeed, the two acts are widely and reasonably regarded as quite distinct. See *Vacco v Quill....* 117 S.Ct., at 2298–2302.[52]

Rehnquist similarly rejected Reinhardt's claim that because how and when to die is an intimate and personal decision, like the decision whether or not to have an abortion, the Court's constitutional protection of the latter liberty interest should extend to the former. That many of the rights and liberties protected by the Due Process clause reflect matters of personal autonomy "does not warrant the conclusion that any and all important, intimate, and personal decisions are so protected ... and *Casey* did not suggest otherwise."[53] Rehnquist then detailed the interests states have in banning all assisted suicide, however personal and intimate the decision for PAS may be: he began these with the interests in protecting human life generally, and preventing suicide specifically, a significant public health issue.

Now that autonomy has been discussed, it is possible to identify the very different thinking represented in the courts by Reinhardt and Rehnquist (and of course those judges who agree with them) on the question of what it is about killing that makes it wrong. Other

---

49. Ibid.
50. Ibid.
51. Ibid., quoting *Compassion in Dying v. State of Washington* (1996).
52. Ibid.
53. Ibid., 2271.

state interests in prohibiting assisted suicide will be taken up in that context.

THE WRONG-MAKING CHARACTERISTICS OF KILLING

On the important question of what makes killing wrong, I wish to remind the reader that Reinhardt did not speak for everyone on the Ninth Circuit Court of Appeals.[54] And, although the U.S. Supreme Court was unanimous in reversing the decision written by Reinhardt for the *en banc* Ninth Circuit Court, there were at least three of the nine justices who did not fully accept Rehnquist's way of framing the issues, while accepting the outcome he reached.[55] The conflict between the special version of Mill and the traditions embedded in current laws and practices on this question is, in any event, most clearly expressed in the opinions written on behalf of the two courts by Reinhardt and Rehnquist.

Reinhardt. What Reinhardt thinks is wrong about killing when it is wrong can be inferred from the reasons he gave for condoning suicide and assisting someone to do it. First of all, an individual should desire death. One can infer from this that it would be wrong, generally,[56] to kill anyone who desires to live or who should be presumed to have such a desire. Secondly, it is not enough that an individual desires death. That desire should be expressed by someone who is terminally ill, suffering from a debilitated, highly dependent state felt to be humiliating or in some way intolerable. (Pain thought to be irremediable is another condition Reinhardt included, but as we saw, that is actually a matter of rejecting total sedation in those instances where nothing short of it suffices to relieve pain.) Under

---

54. There were not only dissenting opinions in response to Reinhardt's opinion, but the first opinion, written by Judge Noonan on behalf of the Ninth Circuit Court, found no constitutional support for a right to PAS. *Compassion in Dying v. State of Washington*, No. 94-35534, 1995 WL 94679 (9th Cir. Mar. 9, 1995).

55. I refer to Justices Breyer, Souter, and Stevens. There is no way to decide from their concurring opinions whether they would or would not agree in full or in part with my analysis of what the Court's opinion, as written by Rehnquist, identifies as the wrong-making characteristics of killing, as found in law, historically and currently.

56. I am using the expression "generally wrong" to accommodate certain exceptions the law makes. For example, it is not a crime, if need be, to kill in self-defense, individually, and, in international law, in defense of a community against aggression, and against those who actually pose the danger, such as members of armed forces. I do not know what other exceptions Reinhardt would make, whether, for example, he would condone capital punishment and, if so, for what crimes.

these conditions the presumption that an individual wishes to live and the state interest in preventing suicide are highly diminished. In these circumstances, one who is terminally ill and expresses a desire to die is presumed to be making a rational request to be assisted in committing suicide. From this one can infer that it would be wrong to kill someone who has some reasonable expectation to enjoy life and to overcome even very grim circumstances. Individuals who express a wish to die when their prospects can be improved to a degree they would recognize as significant may be clinically depressed or temporarily too distressed to make competent judgments. It would be wrong to kill them or fail to prevent them from ending their lives.

Reinhardt expressed great concern with regard to the young people and those of middle age who are committing suicide. He would only permit those who are "near death" to receive the assistance of physicians for the purpose of killing themselves. From this one can infer that it is wrong generally to kill anyone who has a significant length of time to live and has something left to accomplish or live for.

There is a certain vagueness connected to making the obligations to protect life and prevent suicide contingent upon conditions such as being "terminally ill," "humiliating" and "debilitating" life circumstances, and being "near death." Members of the Supreme Court all shared some apprehension about the "slippery slope" that such vagueness invites. Also, the desire to die is very difficult to ascertain with assurance, given the data regarding depression and the frequency with which such desires change when treatment for pain relief and/or depression is pursued. And, as we have discussed previously, those who adhere to a special version of Mill such as Reinhardt espouses give up the presumptions that people naturally seek to preserve their lives. Rehnquist showed no sign of dropping that presumption.

Rehnquist. The presumption that there is a continuous, natural inclination to preserve one's own life was very explicitly present in Rehnquist. Quoting Zephaniah Swift, who became Chief Justice of Connecticut in 1796, he spoke of suicide as "abhorrent to the feelings of mankind, and that strong love of life which is implanted in the human heart...."[57] The original context for this characterization of suicide is this Chief Justice's expression of disapproval

---

57. *Washington v. Glucksberg*, 2264.

of punishing the families of those who commit suicide. Such disapproval was part of a growing consensus at the time. Rehnquist noted that this depiction of suicide clearly indicates that the movement away from the harsh sanctions of the common law did not signify an acceptance of suicide. Note, then, that suicide is described as an act that is contrary to the "strong love of life," a love "implanted in the human heart"; it is contrary to a strong natural and positive disposition toward life or toward living.

Still drawing upon the history of American legal opinions, mostly those found in court opinions, Rehnquist found yet another way in which human beings are continuously and positively attached to their own lives. The right to life is both "sacred" and "inalienable." And, as Rehnquist pointed out, this has two very significant implications: (1) "The consent of a homicide victim is 'wholly immaterial to the guilt of the person who cause[d] [his death]' "; and the prohibitions against assisting suicide never contained exceptions for those "near death," whether because of being "hopelessly diseased," "fatally wounded," or "condemned to death" as criminals. All were "under the protection of law, equally as the lives of those who [were] in the full tide of life's enjoyment, and anxious to continue to live."[58] In other words, the moral and legal obligations of individuals and states to respect and protect life against suicide, assisting in suicide, and criminal homicide generally are not contingent upon either the wish to die or the circumstances that might prompt such a wish. The right to have one's life protected from committing suicide, being assisted in one, or being killed by another, is continuous and equally so for everyone. The worth of that life is "sacred," beyond calculation of the individual's life circumstances.

There is another, closely related way in which the protection of life is continuous and independent of the contingencies that may serve to thwart the desire to continue living. As we observed earlier, the Model Penal Code of 1980 speaks of "the interests in the sanctity of life that are represented by the criminal homicide laws" as "threatened" by anyone "who expresses a willingness to participate in taking the life of another, even though the act may be accomplished with the consent, or at the request, of the suicide vic-

---

58. Ibid., 2265. See also Nigel Cameron, *Death without Dignity: Euthanasia in Perspective* (Edinburgh: Rutherford House Books, 1990).

tim."[59] Not only are individuals to act on the presumption that the protection of life is continuous, but they are to refrain from actions that would undermine the very notion on which life's continuous protection is based, namely, the notion that life has sanctity. Acting on the idea, asserted by Reinhardt, that it sometimes would be cruel and hence wrong to ignore an individual request for assistance to end one's life is viewed in this code as a threat to the "sanctity of life," the very basis in law for prohibiting the taking of life. The worth of life is not regarded as contingent upon calculations of life's prospects and conditions, for such calculations may undermine the natural "love of life" and the natural inalienable claim to have one's life protected from the adverse actions of oneself or of others.

And so, in the legal sources upon which Rehnquist drew, we find the Hobbesian assumptions about human nature and rights: a natural inclination to preserve one's life and, based on that, an inalienable, natural right to life. We find also the Puritan assumptions about human nature and rights: a natural implanted love of life and, based on it, a sacred, inalienable right, suggesting a divine origin for that love of life and the right to its protection. Life's "sanctity" implies also that its worth is for everyone, in whatever circumstances, equally beyond calculation. Reinhardt's assumption of a Millian theological anthropology drops the idea of a natural, continuous pursuit of self-preservation, while retaining the other Hobbesian notion that individuals naturally seek pleasure and avoid pain for themselves. And given that what is right or wrong is based on the calculation of the ratio of pleasure to pain, the worth of life diminishes as pain outweighs pleasure or all pleasure even ceases, and it can become right to end life and wrong to thwart someone from doing so. As we shall observe later, though, Reinhardt neglects aspects of Mill that stress the reasons communities may offer to prohibit the behavior Reinhardt is seeking to exempt from government interference.

Rehnquist, unlike Reinhardt, did not provide a justification for suicide and assisting in it. He does not, therefore, provide any arguments as to when killing in general may be morally justified and legally permitted. We do not know what he thinks about killing in self-defense, whether as an individual or as a member of the armed forces in defense of one's country. But we do not know that about

59. Ibid.

Reinhardt either. Reinhardt did, however, give us some explicit arguments of his own as to when suicide and assisting it should be ethically condoned and legally permitted. What we have from Rehnquist are not his own arguments as to what is wrong about killing oneself or assisting someone to do so. Rather we have from Rehnquist some reasons for legally prohibiting suicide and assisting in a suicide, reasons he selected with approval from legal opinions and practices. These do give us some definite clues as to what goes wrong when an individual commits suicide or aids someone to do so.

First of all, killing is a violation of an individual's right to life; this right is inalienable, and no one should seek to deprive anyone—oneself included—of this right; this right is sacred, and so of continuous, incalculable worth. Depriving oneself or another individual of life is to destroy what is of inestimable worth. A further implication of viewing the right to life as inalienable is that it is wrong to consent to or request to be killed, and it is also wrong to seek such consent.

Secondly, killing is an act directed against a human being's natural, implanted love of life. It is irrational. Rehnquist called attention to the distressed state of at least 95 percent of those who commit suicide. And those who are killed by others or assisted in killing themselves are robbed of their human and humane impulses rather than having these sustained, treated, or otherwise encouraged. Hobbes viewed suicide as irrational, and until recent years being suicidal was universally regarded by medical professionals as a sign of depression in need of medical care. Some still so regard it. Kant viewed suicide as an act that "has no respect for human nature," and declared, "We shrink in horror from suicide because all nature seeks its own preservation."[60] Killing oneself, assisting in a suicide, and killing another individual are quite literally to rob the victim of humanity; these acts are quite literally crimes against humanity, the taking of an innocent life.

Thirdly, Rehnquist has called attention to the symbolic and aspirational aspects of the laws against assisted suicide; these would hold for all the laws governing homicide. Killing oneself, assisting others to do so, and killing others are threats to the sanctity of life. Since it is in the criminal homicide laws that the interests of the

---

60. Immanuel Kant, *Lectures on Ethics*, ed. Benjamin Nelson (New York: Harper & Row, 1963), 150–51.

sanctity of life are represented, as Rehnquist asserted in agreement with the Model Penal Code of 1980, the possibility of protecting the lives of everyone and the very rationale for doing so are threatened or undermined by justifying assisting in a suicide and the act requesting it by considering it a right.[61] Instead of a right, assisted suicide is an act that defies the standard of conduct encompassed by the sanctity of life. In this same context, this norm, the sanctity of life, would also be weakened or undermined by allowing for killing and assisting in a suicide on the basis of the consent and/or the physical or mental conditions of the one who is killed. This would happen because individuals who wish to kill themselves, assist others in doing so, or kill another individual would be acting on the rationale that continued life has no value or at least too little to make it worthwhile. That rationale, in principle, rejects the sanctity of life by failing to apply that standard to all of human life and to all equally. All of this was part of Rehnquist's assertion of the state's "unqualified interest" in protecting individual life, including the interest in preventing suicide.[62]

The whole idea that certain people's lives may no longer be worth living and worthy of the state's protection is a direct threat to the lives of the disabled and terminally ill and undermines their protection "from prejudice, negative and inaccurate stereotypes, and 'societal indifference.' "[63] Rehnquist himself made this point as follows:

> The State's assisted suicide ban reflects and reinforces its policy that the lives of the terminally ill, disabled, and elderly people must be no less valued than the lives of the young and healthy, and that a seriously disabled person's suicidal impulses should be interpreted and treated the same way as anyone else's.[64]

Summary: Reinhardt versus Rehnquist. Reinhardt is willing to justify killing oneself and assisting others to do so when death is desired and life's prospects are such that continuing life is not worthwhile. Both of these justifications for killing are rejected altogether by Rehnquist. Killing oneself, requesting others to help one do so,

---

61. *Washington v. Glucksberg*, 2272.
62. Ibid.
63. Ibid., 2273.
64. Ibid.

helping someone to kill himself or herself, and killing another person are all violations against one's own natural impulses to love life and the standard embedded in criminal law, the sacredness of life. Since the right to life is natural, inalienable, and sacred, the sacredness of life is weakened or undermined by accepting consent to one's death and the contingencies of life as justifications for relinquishing what should be a continuous right: both of these exceptions called for by Reinhardt imply that there are human lives that are not worthy of protection. This is a direct repudiation of the sacredness of life, for it is equally applicable to everyone without discrimination and it is meant to convey that life is of incalculable worth.

HARMFUL EFFECTS OF REINHARDT'S SPECIAL VERSION OF MILL

Reinhardt is part of a development that is unique to America as compared to European nations. His particular version of Mill has found its way into American constitutional law. This development has been thoroughly studied and documented by the American legal scholar Mary Ann Glendon. As she has noted,

> To a greater degree than any other, the American legal system has accepted Mill's version of individual liberty, including its relative inattention to the problem of what may constitute harm to others and unconcern with types of harm that may not be direct and immediate. Indeed, we took Mill's ideas a step further than he did. For, when Mill's ideas about liberty of conduct were taken into American constitutional law, they underwent a sea change. His stern sense of responsibility to family and country, and his decided rejection of any notion that all life-styles were equally worthy of respect, largely dropped out of sight.[65]

It is indeed the case that Reinhardt is quite inattentive to what may be viewed as harm to others. In some instances, he directly eschewed what the Supreme Court considered as harm to others. Through an examination of Reinhardt's treatment of harm to others it will be possible to pinpoint: (1) what of Mill's philosophy he

---

65. Mary Ann Glendon, *Rights Talk: The Impoverishment of Political Discourse* (New York: Free Press, 1991), 72.

neglects or perhaps even misrepresents; (2) the significance of this neglect; and (3) the grounds on which Reinhardt defends himself against the Supreme Court and other possible critics. At the conclusion of this analysis, I will suggest that the neglected aspects of Mill can be used, defended, and assimilated without suppressing other traditions now embedded in law and without engaging in theological debates, implicitly or explicitly. I will argue for this new synthesis, and the framework that supports it, in the next and concluding chapter.

Harm to Others: Euthanasia, Coercion, and Discrimination. Rehnquist, in reversing the decision of the *en banc* Ninth Circuit Court of Appeals to make PAS a constitutional right, considered several ways in which individuals and groups would be harmed by the existence of such a right. One we have just reviewed in the preceding section, namely, discrimination against all who might be considered candidates for PAS and whose lives would be little valued, by reason of being dependent, handicapped, or merely near death in a terminal condition. A second concerns the vulnerability of various groups to "abuse, neglect, and mistakes." These groups include "the poor, the elderly, and the disabled."[66] Rehnquist noted that these groups are at a heightened risk of harm because their autonomy and well-being has already been compromised. Also, to protect against the combination of a bias against the handicapped and a cost-saving mentality requires Washington to ban assisted suicide: "If physician-assisted suicide were permitted many might resort to it to spare their families the substantial financial burden of end-of-life health-care costs."[67] In short, laws against PAS protect the vulnerable from coercion as well as discrimination.

A third kind of harm to others that would accompany a constitutional right to PAS is that there would be a right to suicide that everyone would possess and would be free to exercise. Limiting such a right would, in Rehnquist's view, be very difficult, and permitting suicide, the state may rightly fear, puts one on the path to voluntary and perhaps even involuntary euthanasia. Rehnquist indicated that Reinhardt considerably expanded what is presumably a right possessed only by "competent, terminally ill adults" and only by

---

66. *Washington v. Glucksberg*, 2273. See also Susan Wolf, *Feminism and Bioethics: Beyond Reproduction* (New York: Oxford University Press, 1996).
67. Ibid.

those among them who "wish to hasten their deaths by obtaining medication prescribed by their doctors."[68] Citing Reinhardt's own reasoning, Rehnquist pointed to three instances of broadening the right in question:

> The court noted, for example, that the "decision of a duly appointed surrogate decision maker is for all legal purposes the decision of the patient himself," 79 F3rd, at 832, n. 120; that "in some instances, the patient may be unable to self-administer the drugs and ... administration by the physician ... may be the only way the patient may be able to receive them," id., at 831; and that not only physicians, but also family members and loved ones, will inevitably participate in assisting suicide. Id., at 838, n. 140. [69]

From these assertions by Reinhardt, Rehnquist drew the conclusion that what is alleged to be a limited right to PAS "is likely, in effect, a much broader license, which could prove extremely difficult to police and contain."[70] In a footnote, Rehnquist expressed his conviction that there is a "tendency of a principle to expand itself to the limit of logic," as stated by Justice Cordoza in the context of describing the nature of the judicial process.[71] In the same footnote, Rehnquist also asserted that the court is recognizing "the reasonableness of the widely expressed skepticism about the lack of a principled basis for confining the right."[72]

He backed this up further by reference to what is happening in the Netherlands:

> The Dutch government's own study revealed that in 1990 there were 2,300 cases of voluntary euthanasia (defined as "the deliberate termination of another's life at his request"), 400 cases of assisted suicide, and more than 1,000 cases of euthanasia without an explicit request. In addition to these latter 1,000 cases, the study found ... 4,941 cases where physicians

---

68. Ibid., 2274.
69. Ibid.
70. Ibid.
71. Ibid., footnote 23.
72. Ibid. At this point, Rehnquist also refers to briefs submitted to the Court as well as other sources. One such source, the AMA's *Report of the Council on Ethical and Judicial Affairs* asserts: "[I]f assisted suicide is permitted, then there is a strong argument for allowing euthanasia."

administered lethal morphine overdoses without the patients' explicit consent.[73]

Since euthanasia is supposed to be voluntary, this study reveals abuses despite government regulations in place. Furthermore, the practice has not been limited to competent, terminally ill adults who are suffering physically; there have been cases involving severely disabled neonates and elderly persons suffering from dementia.[74] Reinhardt is aware of the arguments and studies that Rehnquist used to warn of the harms associated with and risked by permitting PAS. From one perspective, namely, his use of Millian consequentialist arguments to conflate comfort-only care and PAS, none of Rehnquist's concerns are germane or convincing. After all, comfort-only care is already ethically and legally accepted. Whatever risks of harm attach to PAS as a means of hastening death attach as well to hastening death by means of comfort-only care. Specifically, Reinhardt argued that "the recognition of any right creates the possibility of abuse."[75] He dismissed the studies of what is happening in the Netherlands on the grounds that these studies are interpreted differently by various scholars and what is happening there may not be relevant to the American situation.[76]

With respect to possible medical mistakes that may be made, Reinhardt is so committed to the individual calculus that justifies PAS, he said that "should an error actually occur it is likely to benefit the individual by permitting a victim of unmanageable pain and suffering to end his life peacefully and with dignity at the time he deems most desirable."[77] This same strong commitment led him to say of the lack of access to medical care associated with poverty that the poor will be less likely than others to have the opportunity to enjoy the benefits of PAS. That should be a concern rather than the

---

73. Ibid.

74. Ibid. Rehnquist cites additional studies. See also footnote 64 in chap. 2 of this book.

75. *Compassion in Dying v. State of Washington* (1996), 831. Reinhardt also argues that *Roe v. Wade* was supposed to create horrific consequences that have not materialized. That is ironic because one of the predicted consequences was that advocacy of PAS and euthanasia would follow. Reinhardt does not mention this prediction.

76. Ibid., 830.

77. Ibid., 824.

fear that a disproportionate number of the poor will be among those who receive PAS because of any special vulnerability to coercion.[78]

THE SUPPRESSION OF OTHER TRADITIONS

How can Reinhardt justify his version of the Millian tradition, or, as he put it, "Millsian principles," while setting aside the whole tradition of natural rights and the synthesis supporting it, embedded in the founding documents and laws of the United States? Remember that Reinhardt claimed that his decision is based on facts and law. To begin with, he used a consequentialist (Millian) mode of moral reasoning to reach the conclusion that PAS is no different ethically and constitutionally from comfort-only care. The latter, he argued, has been sanctioned by courts in a way that grants a constitutionally protected right to hasten one's death. So, factually, logically, and by law, PAS and refusing or terminating medical treatment should enjoy the same status in law. The conflation of PAS and refusing or terminating life-sustaining medical treatment is a debated mode of reasoning in ethics. Reinhardt did not treat it as a philosophical debate, however, but as a fact of life and/or a correct way of reasoning logically. That way of seeing things allowed Reinhardt to draw on existing law with respect to comfort-only care to make his case for legalizing PAS, oblivious to any alternative modes of moral reasoning.

Secondly, Reinhardt sought to justify his version of Mill as applied to PAS by characterizing the decision it enables him to reach as morally and religiously neutral, leaving individuals of various persuasions free to follow their beliefs. But he did not regard the opinion of those who disagree with him as neutral. As he said, rather emphatically,

> Under our constitutional system, neither the state nor the majority of the people can impose its will upon the individual in a matter so highly "central to personal dignity and autonomy.... " Those who believe strongly that death must come without physician assistance are free to follow that creed, be they doctors or patients. They are not free, however, to force their views, their religious convictions or their

78. Ibid., 825.

philosophies on all the other members of a democratic society, and to compel those whose values differ with theirs to die painful, protracted, and agonizing deaths.[79]

Previously we saw that Reinhardt treated his opinion on a philosophically debated issue as if it were a fact, or at least obviously correct. Now he is treating those who draw on traditions other than his version of Mill as willing to impose their will and beliefs on others, doing so rather cruelly on those suffering near the end of their lives. He either did not see, or chose not to see, how he not only is imposing on the thinking and behavior of others, but also blocking from the continuous shaping of laws, constitutional and legislative, traditions that have a long enduring place in forming and sustaining such laws. In this case, the traditions that are thwarted are those that regard assisting in a suicide as a violation of human rights, of the natural right to life and the rights to any further liberty and possible happiness.

How could Reinhardt think that he achieved a morally and religiously neutral standpoint? Certainly he was not showing any awareness that he was implicitly adhering to a theological anthropology, a doctrine of human nature shared by Mill: human beings naturally seek their own pleasure and avoid pain for themselves. By allowing individuals to make their own calculations of their own pleasure and pain and allowing them to act on these calculations, individuals may see PAS as right for them and choose it, or wrong for them, and reject it. This hidden doctrine of human nature was evident when he claimed that

> by permitting the *individual* to exercise the right to *choose* we are following the constitutional mandate to take such decisions out of the hands of the government, both state and federal, and to put them where they rightly belong, in the hands of the people.[80]

Circuit Judge Fernandez, writing in dissent of the majority opinion written by Reinhardt, had a different reaction to issues that divide philosophers and others and a different interpretation of what it means to put an issue in the hands of the people. Having declared

---

79. Ibid., 839.
80. Ibid.

that there is no constitutional right to commit suicide, he made the following observation:

> The arguments for and against suicide raise an issue which would elicit competing responses from even our most well trained philosophers. Like so many other issues, it is one "for the people to decide." [Reference omitted] Our constitution leaves it to them. It is they and their representatives who must grapple with the riddle and solve it.[81]

Like other dissenting judges of the Ninth Circuit Court, and later the unanimous Supreme Court, Fernandez ascribed to the elected representatives the responsibility to forge policies that protect human life. His assumption was that all of the people have a stake in sustaining life, and the fact that some people may wish to die under some circumstances does not by itself make the case for a policy to accommodate such wishes. What that would mean for all of the people should be examined. An elected body representing all of the people is the locus for Fernandez, as well as other dissenting judges and the Supreme Court; in this body the moral bases for laws applying to a whole people are to be debated and decided. Such a body is also beholden to the electorate when policies are indeed perceived to be less than satisfactorily protective of innocent human life. In short, whether someone is permitted to assist in a suicide is not a private matter, but rather a public matter of creating and enforcing laws that apply to everyone. One way to state the divide between Reinhardt and these dissenters on the Ninth Circuit Court is to note that Reinhardt has advocated the privatization of an area that would substantially change the laws against homicide: the principle in law is that "the consent of a homicide victim is wholly immaterial to the guilt of the person who cause[d] [his death]. . . . "[82]

Now I can explain why I have repeatedly referred to Reinhardt's views as a "version of Mill." He gives us Mill without attending to Mill's moral criterion "the greatest good for the greatest number"; he gives us Mill without attending to what Mill calls "moral rules," essential to everyone's well-being and essential to the security of whole societies.[83] It is not at all clear that Mill would accept

---

81. Ibid., Fernandez, J., dissenting, 857.
82. *Washington v. Glucksberg*, 2265.
83. John Stuart Mill, "Utilitarianism," in *The Philosophy of John Stuart Mill*, ed. Marshall Cohen (New York: Random House, 1961), 391.

PAS. What is relatively certain is that Mill would, if he were to be consistent in his thinking, weigh the consequences of permitting assisted suicide insofar as they affect the efficacy and sustenance of the moral rules essential to communal life. Undermining these rules would be very harmful indeed. Reinhardt has not done this explicitly. He could argue that his review of state interests, and his arguments that these would not be undermined by a constitutional right to PAS, constitute attention to this aspect of the impact of his decision. However, he has so weakened the state interest in life near its end and so heightened the individual interest in the liberty to end it that his conclusion is already found in these claims, based on his own "personal" calculus of what makes life worth living. What is more, his version of Mill is not acknowledged to be what it is—his own moral or social rule, one he expects everyone to accept. In privatizing beliefs about when life is worth living, he has either taken assisting in a suicide, at least in some circumstances, out of the realm of morality, or rendered utterly subjective moral judgments regarding such a practice.

Unlike the Puritans and the biblical and classical philosophical traditions undergirding them, Reinhardt does not have a social concept of the self. When all are to be free to act on their beliefs about when to hasten death, he believes the decision is then in the hands of the "people." The people, in this instance, are individuals unconnected by a common moral basis for making laws that would prevent individuals from assisting in suicides. But not everyone would be free to follow his or her consciences had Reinhardt prevailed. Indeed, the *people* would not be free. They would not be free to retain the laws now prevailing with regard to assisted suicide, and they would not be free to prevent suicide in some circumstances. Indeed, a whole area would no longer be in the hands of the representatives and deliberative bodies representing all of the people. Reinhardt's hidden theological anthropology provides no clearly natural basis for a common morality or for democratic deliberative bodies. The social concept of the self, shared by the classical philosophers of Greece and Rome and Jewish and Christian philosophers and theologians, posits a natural basis for the moral knowledge necessary for communal living and democratic structures, a natural basis to be examined in the next chapter. The modern philosophies of natural rights, as in Hobbes and Locke, hold governments to be morally beholden to the protection of natural rights, including the right to life; these they saw as rights that could not and should not be relinquished in any social contract establishing a government. Reinhardt's theology as reflected in his opinion opposed and suppressed these traditions, seemingly without any consciousness that he was doing so. Nor did he even consider as harm the suppression of the traditions that may be essential to a common morality, as expressed so far in the "sanctity of life" to which our criminal homicide laws appeal and which they embody.

THE NEED FOR A SYNTHETIC APPROACH

The various judges on our courts are disagreeing with one another over the issue of whether to permit, as legal, the practice of PAS. They are not convinced by one another's arguments. A major reason for this are hidden assumptions: about human nature—theological or philosophical anthropologies—and about the proper modes of moral reasoning. This can be seen in so vital a question as the very basis for regarding killing as wrong when it is so to be regarded, legally and morally.

One cannot simply rest content to assert the opinions expressed by Rehnquist, even if they were to be widely accepted by the public. There are and will be judges who shape and form their opinions in accord with the special version of Mill so clearly exemplified by the reasoning of Judge Reinhardt. What is equally important is that Rehnquist, quite appropriately, relied for his arguments on facts and opinions from legal sources and sources he considers to have legal weight, such as the AMA on the ethics of the medical profession. From a philosophical standpoint, this constitutes an appeal to authority rather than a bona fide philosophical case for one's opinion. Mounting such a philosophical argument would not be appropriate for a constitutional court, not, at least, in the judgment of Chief Justice Rehnquist and those who share his method of constitutional analysis.

But all of this creates what I regard as a very serious problem. There are those judges like Judge Reinhardt who are not at all shy about introducing into the reasoning of their courts explicit philosophical arguments reflecting a special version of Mill, and one which suppresses other modes of moral reasoning and also other moral standards now present in law and social practices. All of this is done with hidden premises as their basis, premises that are not exposed in the courts either by the proponents of PAS or by its opponents. The problem with such arguments is that they ignore existing moral traditions that have long proved viable in sustaining democratic structures, communal life, and individual rights. To replace this current synthesis of moral traditions with this special version of Mill is to introduce a considerable social experiment the viability of which is at best untested and at worst unable adequately to protect and sustain individual and communal life.

In the concluding chapter, I will address this problem by examining what best protects and sustains individual and communal life. Through this examination, a new synthesis may be forged, which relies on the Natural Rights Synthesis as well as drawing on a wider view of Mill's thought than the special version of Mill employed by those arguing for the legalization of assisted suicide. As we will see, the values that form the foundation of this new synthesis are best upheld by prohibiting assisted suicide.

4

Moral Underpinnings
of a Synthetic Approach

AS OUR PREVIOUS CHAPTERS have revealed, there is a special version of a moral tradition fashioned out of the philosophy of John Stuart Mill strongly asserting itself in U.S. courts. Judge Reinhardt provided a strong expression of this thinking in the opinion he wrote for the Ninth Circuit Court of Appeals.[1] Since the moral and theological traditions currently found in our laws and democratic processes have proved viable, in the sense of sustaining themselves, but, even more importantly, viable in the sense of sustaining a robust, communal life, there is a question about the relatively new kid on the block—the special version of Mill—a mostly twentieth-century entry. The question is whether such a truncated version of Mill provides sustenance for the norms that sustain our laws, our democratic institutions, our individual lives, and our communal life as such. Being portrayed as disconnected individuals with incompatible views on grave matters of life and death at the very least

---

1. *Compassion in Dying v. State of Washington,* 793rd 790 (9th Cir. 1996). In chap. 3, I documented a description of the power and sweep of this special version of Mill published in 1890 by Samuel D. Warren and Louis D. Brandeis, "The Right to Privacy," *Harvard Law Review,* no. 4 (1890), in which they asserted that the "right to life has come to mean the right to enjoy life,—the right to be let alone" (193). Later, in 1928, Justice Brandeis called the "right to be let alone the most comprehensive of rights, and the right most valued by civilized men" (in *Olmstead v. United States,* 277 U.S. 438, 48 S.Ct. 564, 72 L. Ed. 944 [1928], 478 and 48 S.Ct., 572, Brandeis, J., dissenting). For Reinhardt, this is the "second most famous dissent in American jurisprudence," and he noted that the words of Brandeis have been fully quoted "in several opinions of the Court," meaning the Supreme Court, and "innumerable appellate court decisions." *Compassion in Dying v. State of Washington,* 800. Notice how this "right to be let alone" suppresses the natural rights tradition, specifically the right to life, a right considered the most basic and most to be prized by Hobbes.

deserves scrutiny. And that is what I propose to do in this concluding chapter. I will give reasons why I think basing law on this special version of Mill is not sufficient for nurturing and protecting individual lives and communities; as a social experiment, it would be fraught with dangers.

Happily, Mill actually shares the concern I am expressing about the basis on which individuals and communities can and should be sustained. Attending to his notion of justice as it relates to moral rules essential to the very existence of societies, one can draw on Mill in a way that does not conflict with the Natural Rights Synthesis. Furthermore, doing so avoids the need for courts and legislatures to conduct full debates over what doctrine of human nature to adopt. This important debate is best left to ongoing public debates and those that have been carried on by philosophers and theologians for centuries. How judges and legislators are shaped by their views of human nature remains important, for reasons that will be made apparent. However, public policy has open to it a shared morality, a synthesis of moral traditions, the nature of which does not have to be determined each time by the outcome of a debate over human nature.

And so in the concluding chapter I wish to offer a framework for thinking about the very kinds of human relationships that are absolutely requisite to the nurturance, protection, and continuation of our individual and communal existence. These would not be invented, but identified and defended. They are, and long have been, sustaining our individual and communal existence. As it will turn out, these requisites of individual and communal life are best nourished by prohibiting, rather than permitting, assisted suicide in general and PAS in particular.

One can agree that the special version of Mill in the courts is problematic in just the way I have stated but remain relatively unconcerned, at least for now. Why? Because one believes that this whole way of reasoning, and the conclusions reached by it, have been decisively rejected and refuted by the opinions Chief Justice Rehnquist wrote for a unanimous Supreme Court.[2] Indeed, that is precisely what James Bopp and Richard E. Coleson maintain when they say of Rehnquist's opinions that they "reveal that all the argu-

---

2. *Washington v. Glucksberg*, 117 S.Ct. 2558 (1997); *Vacco v. Quill*, 117 S.Ct. 2293 (1997).

ments and situations have been considered in the decided cases."[3] They characterize the United States Supreme Court's rulings as a "stunning defeat" for proponents of legalized assisted suicide, a defeat that

> means that the future efforts by assisted suicide advocates to find protection for PAS in state constitutions or to enact laws legalizing assisted suicide by legislation will be heavily burdened by the U.S. Supreme Court's reasoned rejection of the assisted suicide movement's best arguments. One by one the High Court analyzed the claims presented by able advocates . . . and found them unconvincing.[4]

In the light of all this, Bopp and Coleson are convinced that another case, brought before the U.S. Supreme Court, "would not bring a different result absent a failure of stare decisis on the Court. [Footnote omitted] The federal constitutional battle is over, at least for this generation."[5]

But it is not a certainty that the U.S. Supreme Court would abide by its present decisions were its membership to change. And that could happen before this generation is past. There are now, and will be in the future, judges who share Reinhardt's philosophical outlook and hidden theological premises. Furthermore, as we have seen, there is philosophical support for the arguments that favor PAS and even euthanasia. Rehnquist's opinions relied on the authority of past legal rulings and on the interpretations he and other jurists gave of these rulings. And though he cited sources that contained philosophical arguments, he did not provide arguments as to why these sources and past decisions, and the moral traditions they represent, should persist over against the special version of Mill and its alleged moral and religious neutrality. For some jurists and philosophers, it is this alleged neutrality that makes Reinhardt's framework and viewpoint superior to those he and others see as based on moral and religious views, views that should not be legally enforced against the wishes and beliefs of individuals who do not share those views and the traditions on which they are based. Bopp and Coleson do not address this clash of traditions, nor the fact that Reinhardt defends the

---

3. James Bopp and Richard E. Coleson, "Three Strikes: Is an Assisted Suicide Right?" *Issues in Law and Medicine* 15, no. 1 (Summer 1999): 5.
4. Ibid.
5. Ibid.

superiority of his philosophical outlook without a comparable defense by Rehnquist of the traditions he invokes as those which now, and for more than seven hundred years, are embedded in law and still govern the current laws against homicide generally and suicide in particular. What is more, in the absence of raising doubts about the viability of this special version of Mill, judges and lawyers now and in the future will still have reasons, and philosophical defenders of such reasons, to approve PAS as a constitutional right and/or to influence others to adopt PAS as a right guaranteed by state laws. Nor have those who may be inclined to adopt this special version of Mill been given any reasons, at least not explicitly, why they should recognize that Mill's corpus provides concepts and modes of thinking such that accepting them could lead to drawing some of the same conclusions contained in the U.S. Supreme Court decisions regarding PAS. In any event, Bopp and Coleson notwithstanding, the proponents of PAS, whether judges or philosophers, are not persuaded by appeals to existing moral and legal traditions that do not give them explicit reasons for giving up their own presumed morally and religiously neutral stance as the basis for legalizing PAS. As far as they are concerned, no one opposed to PAS has to request it, and no physician has to practice it. At the same time, anyone whose moral and religious beliefs condone PAS under certain circumstances should not have their individual moral and religious beliefs suppressed by law when they wish to act on those beliefs.

But this is not a morally and religiously neutral stance as alleged. Were PAS to be legalized, those who believe that every suicide should be prevented if possible would not be permitted by law to prevent those suicides and those instances of assisting in them that are regarded as lawful. Their moral and religious beliefs would be suppressed by law.

There is no way to avoid the issue on which Reinhardt and Rehnquist differed: what makes killing wrong when it is wrong. Reinhardt regards PAS as morally defensible and as a practice the law is obligated to permit; Rehnquist does not. On what grounds can Rehnquist defend his view that assisting in a suicide undermines the sacredness of life, the very basis of the laws against homicide? Reinhardt does not think that permitting PAS would have this or any other harmful effect morally or legally. He is well aware that the law invokes the sacredness of life. If he is to be persuaded to adopt Rehnquist's position, Reinhardt will need to have reasons that convince him he should do so. It is not enough to assert that the practice stands in violation of life's sacredness. As Ronald Dworkin has argued, the whole debate about euthanasia is not about the sacredness of human life; rather it is the case that

> ...most people treat living as a sacred responsibility, and this responsibility seems most intense when they contemplate death, their own or someone else's. People who want an early peaceful death, for themselves or their relatives, are not rejecting or denigrating the sanctity of life; on the contrary, they believe that a quicker death shows more respect for life than a protracted one... both sides in the debate about euthanasia share a concern for life's sanctity; they are united by that value, and disagree only about how best to interpret and respect it.[6]

Because people disagree about how to interpret and respect life's sanctity, Dworkin, like Reinhardt, claims that there should be a constitutional right to decide for ourselves as individuals when our lives should end.

This chapter begins, then, with what it is that makes killing wrong when it is wrong. Or, to put it another way, the chapter begins by seeking to discover whether there are or are not compelling reasons to consider suicide and assisting in it as actions that the law should seek to prevent, even in the circumstances put forward by Reinhardt, Dworkin, and other judges and philosophers. It will prove necessary to discuss how autonomy is to be understood, since respect for autonomy is at the heart of the argument that those who choose death are not bound by anyone who permits or enables someone to make that choice. Furthermore, since those who hold to the special version of Mill, espoused by Reinhardt and other jurists, do not consider PAS as a harmful practice were it to be implemented, it is important to consider what possible harms Mill himself would have been led to consider relative to proposals to legalize PAS. As I wish to argue, laws against suicide are compatible with the Millian tradition considered as a whole. This more com-

6. Ronald Dworkin, *Life's Dominion: An Argument about Abortion, Euthanasia, and Individual Freedom* (New York: Random House, 1994), 238. Although Dworkin at this point is talking about euthanasia, his position on PAS, as will be noted later, is based on this same argument favoring voluntary euthanasia. See also John Spier, *Who Owns Our Bodies? Making Moral Choices in Health Care* (New York: Radcliffe Medical Press, 1977).

prehensive version of that tradition could forge a synthesis with the traditions of mutual responsibilities and natural rights now embedded in our laws. This could be accomplished without coming to an agreement with respect to the differing theological anthropologies lodged within these traditions. These are the matters I will need to discuss in order to make a case for continuing to ban assisted suicide.

What I will be arguing in this concluding chapter is that: (1) there is a moral structure that supports Rehnquist's view of what is harmful about the act of killing and assisting someone to commit such an act; (2) this moral structure would be threatened or undermined by legalizing PAS; (3) there are elements in Mill's thinking that lend support to the preceding two contentions. If jurists were to work with these elements in Mill's thinking, they could forge and work with a new synthesis of all the most significant and influential traditions that now shape American law.

THE MORAL REQUISITES OF INDIVIDUAL AND COMMUNAL LIFE

In the previous chapter, we saw that Judge Reinhardt asserted the view that there is nothing morally wrong with killing oneself, and requesting a physician's assistance to do so, for individuals who desire death, are near death, are terminally ill and experiencing permanent, irremediable suffering, or are under circumstances felt to be humiliating or in some way intolerable. The wrongfulness of killing, on this view, is made contingent upon the desire to live and the circumstances of one's life, particularly the anticipated length of one's life and some degree of freedom from undue suffering. These contingencies are somewhat vague and elastic, and they do raise the common concerns over containing any law permitting some such deaths. Reinhardt expects the states to be able to set out and enforce limits to permissible instances of assisted suicide, but other judges are dubious.[7] As we saw in the previous chapter as well, the Supreme Court found that Reinhardt's reasoning allowed for what

7. In a recent test of Alaska's law, Judge Eric T. Sanders cites the data used in *Glucksberg* regarding the difficulties of regulating and containing the practice of PAS: he ruled that Alaska's ban of PAS does not violate Alaska's constitution, *Kevin Sampson v. State of Alaska* (September 9, 1999), reprinted in full in *Issues in Law and Medicine* 15, no. 2 (Fall 1999): 199–219.

would amount to euthanasia in circumstances "difficult to police and contain."[8] And, furthermore, Rehnquist does not think that Reinhardt can provide a "principled basis" for confining a right to PAS.[9]

But Reinhardt and others who do not think that there is a morally significant difference between comfort-only care and PAS, insofar as both can be construed as hastening death, are not persuaded by these alleged difficulties about containing a right to PAS. Whatever concerns may obtain with regard to PAS, such as the risks of error, coercion, discrimination, and overstepping of the boundaries set by law, may obtain as well with regard to the right to choose comfort-only care already legally permitted. If, therefore, one is to decide between the views of Reinhardt and Rehnquist, it is necessary to take up the question of what makes killing wrong when it is wrong. How one answers that question determines how one answers the question of whether comfort-only care and PAS should or should not be morally distinguished. Beauchamp and Childress, as we noted in chapter 2, answer that question in a way that supports the view they share with Reinhardt, that comfort-only care insofar as it hastens death is not morally distinguishable or, at least not significantly so, from PAS and voluntary euthanasia.

According to Beauchamp and Childress, what is wrong about causing someone's death is that the one who is killed suffers a harm or loss; it is not wrong because of losses that others encounter.

> What makes it [causing death] wrong, when it is wrong, is that a person is harmed—that is, suffers a setback to interests that the person otherwise would not have experienced. In particular one is caused the loss of the capacity to plan and choose a future, together with a deprivation of expectable goods. This explains why inflicting death both harms and wrongs a person.[10]

From this line of reasoning, Beauchamp and Childress conclude that, for an individual who "desires death rather than life's more typical goals and projects . . . causing that person's death at his or

---

8. *Washington v. Glucksberg*, 2274.
9. Ibid., footnote 23.
10. Tom Beauchamp and James F. Childress, *Principles of Biomedical Ethics*, 4th ed. (New York: Oxford University Press, 1994), 236.

her autonomous request does not either harm or wrong the person."[11] Whether one arranges for death by refusing treatment or by requesting PAS, the fact that death is willed, that is, knowingly chosen, means that those who in either instance cause death have harmed no one. For Beauchamp and Childress, PAS and active, voluntary euthanasia do not differ in this regard, and so are morally and legally justifiable. The key ingredients that justify arranging for one's death, whether by refusing life-sustaining treatment, PAS, or euthanasia, are that the one whose death it is freely requests the arrangement and so is not harmed. Indeed, Beauchamp and Childress argue that patients are harmed in certain very burdensome circumstances if PAS is not legally permitted and no one honors their requests for aid to end their lives. Since patients who will very soon die when treatment is removed do have their right to autonomy honored, the failure to grant the same right to lingering patients requesting PAS in equally unbearable circumstances "seems tantamount to condemning the patient to live a life he or she does not want."[12]

There are two things Beauchamp and Childress say individuals stand to lose when they lose their lives: (1) the capacity to plan and choose a future; (2) life's more typical goods and projects. These losses are the harms that make killing wrong when it is wrong. But, on this view, if individuals no longer want the capacity to plan and choose a future, the loss of this capacity is not a harm. And if individuals do not want any more of the goods expected from continuing to live, the loss of them is also not a harm. Beauchamp and Childress do not posit human life itself as a good, and certainly not as an inalienable right. Rather, life is a right only if individuals desire and claim it; life is good only as a means to whatever individuals regard as good.

Now Beauchamp and Childress might want to interrupt the discussion at this point to remind us that the context in which they are speaking about individuals as being condemned to lives they may not wish to live is one of dying under very undesirable, even intolerable, circumstances. However, it is fair to ask whether it is the perspective of such individuals that is to prevail or that of others. If, as Beauchamp and Childress claim, autonomy is the key reason for

11. Ibid.
12. Ibid., 226.

granting individuals legal permission to request PAS and euthanasia, then it should be the perceptions of those who regard their own lives as intolerable that should prevail. After all, individuals are not harmed if and when they no longer desire their capacities to plan and choose a future and no longer desire any of life's typical goods and projects. Beauchamp and Childress do not provide a reason to say to such individuals, given that they are competent, "you ought to desire to live when you are not terminally ill, not in physical pain, and not in any way debilitated." They could presume that, absent such maladies, people would not commit suicide. But they should not so presume, and probably do not, for they undoubtedly know the facts are otherwise. It is more likely that Beauchamp and Childress, like Judge Reinhardt, are simply trying to carve out a sphere in which autonomy reigns, a sphere comparable to that enjoyed by those whose death can be hastened by refusing life-sustaining treatment when they are terminally ill and near death. However, they do so without offering a principled reason for preventing suicides. In principle, the only reason they give is that people should not be killed, or assisted in killing themselves, because they express no wish to have this happen. Beauchamp and Childress do not give us a reason why, under some circumstances at least, individuals ought to have no desire to kill themselves or be killed.

Beauchamp and Childress could take the view, expressed by some philosophers, that you try to prevent suicides generally because the individuals being rescued from death will be grateful.[13] The premise of such rescues could be that the circumstances in which such individuals find themselves are such that it is reasonable to consider their despair temporary and amenable to change: they are not terminally ill, near death, and suffering in ways and to a degree they find intolerable and irremediable. If they were in such conditions, Beauchamp and Childress would grant them the legal freedom and moral right to PAS and euthanasia. But that means that there is no moral justification for what hospice care was designed to do and does so well, namely, prevent suicide and euthanasia.

---

13. Ronald Dworkin, Thomas Nagel, Robert Nozick, John Rawls, Thomas Scanlon, and Judith Jarvis Thomson expressed this view in an amicus curiae brief submitted to the Supreme Court for its consideration of PAS. It was published as "Assisted Suicide: The Philosophers' Brief," in *New York Review*, March 27, 1997, 41–47. This brief is published in full in *Issues in Law and Medicine* 15, no. 2 (Fall 1999): 183–98. Hereafter, references to this brief will be this journal and its pages, identified as "Brief of Ronald Dworkin et al."

Hospice physicians repeatedly report, and studies show, that once they provide comfort-only care, the patients who expressed a desire to end their lives, or have them ended, change their minds, or else no longer pursue ending their lives as an option.[14] Strictly speaking, Beauchamp and Childress have posited situations in which attempts to change a patient's desire for immediate death is morally wrong, even reprehensible. However, the situations they posit as unchangeable cannot, and will not, be changed unless the attempt is made to change such situations. The question, then, remains: is there any moral justification for providing comfort-only care and not PAS or euthanasia when requested, in the face of conditions that patients, at the time of such intervention, have reason to regard as hopelessly undesirable?

As we noted in chapter 3, Rehnquist found reasons in law for denying a right to be assisted in a suicide. These are reasons as well that killing is wrong when it is wrong. We identified the following three: (1) killing is the violation of an individual's inalienable right to life; (2) killing irrationally runs counter to a human being's natural love of life; and (3) killing oneself, assisting others to do so, and killing others violate the sanctity of life and threaten adherence to it. Can these reasons for the wrongfulness of killing be morally justified as they have so far been justified within law? I want now to suggest why I think they can be.

The Inalienable Right to Life. In the legal reasoning Rehnquist drew upon, the right to life was described as both sacred and inalienable. The idea of the sacredness or sanctity of life I wish to take up below. For now, the focus will be on the right to life as natural and as an inalienable endowment of individual human beings as such. I will not begin with definitions of "natural" and "inalienable" but rather say what these mean at the conclusion of an extended argument that is intended to make a case for speaking of life as a right of every individual, and as a right that is both natural and inalienable. I will not be content to regard this right, so described, as a self-evident truth. Hopefully, the reader will come to appreciate why it was nevertheless reasonable for those signing the American Declaration of Independence so to regard the right to life.

---

14. See, for example, Robert G. Twycross, "Where there is hope, there is life: a view from the hospice," in *Euthanasia Examined: Ethical, Clinical, and Legal Perspectives*, ed. John Keown (Cambridge: Cambridge University Press, 1995), 141–68. See the many cases, studies, and publications cited by Twycross.

The contemporary moral philosopher Alan Gewirth has constructed a strong defense of natural human rights.[15] He begins with the notion that morality is concerned with actions. Seeking to base moral claims on reason and not upon utility or contingent desires or attitudes, he asks what is logically necessary for human agents to achieve by their actions any of their purposes whatsoever. This he identifies as freedom and well-being. They are the procedural and substantive conditions necessary to pursue and achieve the goods agents seek. The objects of rights, what one has a right to, are not these goods sought through purposive actions but rather the freedom and well-being required as conditions for pursuing human purposes as such, as well as chances of success in achieving the purposes of human actions. The right to life is included as a basic right within the overall right to well-being.[16] Rights are moral, for Gewirth, because they are "based upon" or justifiable through a valid moral principle; a principle is "moral" in that it identifies the categorically obligatory nature of certain requirements of action. These requirements are equally requirements for all actual or prospective agents and serve important interests all persons or recipients equally share. No individual can logically claim these rights from others without granting that others can, on the same basis, claim these same rights from them.

But Gewirth has not completely and consistently followed his own method of explicating the logically necessary, universal conditions for human agency. He takes autonomous individuals as his starting point: the necessary conditions for pursuing and achieving an individual's purposes as an agent identify our moral rights, namely, freedom and well-being, including life. What Gewirth has not considered is what is necessary, logically and functionally, for there to be agents at all. He portrays agents without regard to the fact that they cease and come to be: agents can neither come to be nor persist on their own. Human agents only exist because of the cooperative behavior of other human agents. To begin with, human beings come to be through procreation and persist through

---

15. Alan Gewirth, *Reason and Morality* (Chicago: University of Chicago Press, 1978), and *Human Rights: Essays on Justification and Applications* (Chicago: University of Chicago Press, 1982).

16. For a discussion of what Gewirth means by characterizing the right to life as "basic," see Gewirth, *Reason and Morality*, 211–19. Life as a right is sometimes absolute (see *Human Rights*, 233).

nurture, instruction, and a whole array of actions, practices, and agencies that protects human life. There are then certain proclivities that make human life possible at all: the proclivities to procreate and nurture it. There are other proclivities that are essential to the continuation of a human life: the proclivities to nurture and protect life. Then there are as well certain inhibitions essential to the continuation of a human life: the inhibitions against killing, against taking away or failing to provide the necessities of life, and against lying, a practice that would undermine the whole network, social, legal, and educational, that protects human life. All of these proclivities and inhibitions, and the individual and group behavior they make possible, also are requisite for the realization of human freedom. The individual freedom to pursue one's purposes can be undermined or thwarted by a lack of nurture and instruction, or by lying, or by stealing, or ultimately by being killed or killing oneself.

Human rights then cannot simply be rendered actual by claiming them or by asserting or proving their necessity for achieving our individual purposes. Human rights become actual only through actions, patterns of behavior, and social arrangements that render their actualization possible. I cannot come to be by claiming it as a right. I came to be by the loving procreative, nurturant, and life-protecting behavior of my parents and of the social and legal entities in the community in which my parents lived. My life persisted because the proclivities and inhibitions protecting life persisted in the behavior of my parents and members of my larger community.[17] For these same reasons, my life and the lives of all other individual human beings now persist. For these same reasons communities come to be and exist, no community can come to be, or continue to exist, without some procreation and nurture of life, and without behavior that accords with the inhibitions against killing, lying, and stealing. These behaviors and behavioral constraints constitute morally significant relations between and among individuals and groups.[18] What, then, does it mean to assert that human rights be-

---

17. As I am using the term "community," families as well as nations and their subdivisions can qualify as communities: "A community is *an affiliated and mutually beneficial network of interdependent human beings who, as human beings, share what is requisite for forming and sustaining such a network.*" Arthur J. Dyck, *Rethinking Rights and Responsibilities: The Moral Bonds of Community* (Cleveland: Pilgrim Press, 1994), 126. Each key term in this definition is explained on pages 126 and 127.

18. Another morally significant relation, a requisite of familial life and nurture of

come actual through the behavior patterns that create and sustain these morally significant relations, behavior I will henceforth call morally responsible?

To begin with, behaving in these morally responsible ways is exhibited by and expected from individuals and communities. These behaviors are "natural" both in the sense of being actual or real, and in the sense of being a continuous, predictable set of occurrences. They evoke expectations. Having brought a child into being, nurtured, educated, and protected it, parents expect, even seek similar proclivities and inhibitions in that child. In turn, other members of any larger community expect that parents will be morally responsible, that is, provide for the nurture, education, and necessities of life for the child they spawned. Indeed, their expectations are such that it is appropriate to say that the child has a right to the necessities of life, a right to life. Should the parents fail to meet these expectations by threatening this right, the right of the child to life will become a right claimed on behalf of that child by the community through its legally authorized agencies to try to assure that the right is not violated. Parents may even lose custody of that child so that others will be free to meet the moral responsibilities owed the child and thereby prevent the violation of its rights. Needless to say irresponsible behavior that results in death is subject to legal punishments on those who violated the child's right to life.

Rights, then, exist continuously as expectations that our natural moral responsibilities, requisite to our existence as living human beings, will be met. Given the continuity of these moral requisites of human agency, individually and communally, we are not usually any more conscious of these expectations than we are of the law of gravity that also is a requisite of all of our activities on this earth. But when any of these moral responsibilities requisite to our freedom, our well-being, or our very lives are not met, expectations tend to turn into claims on behalf of the one who is threatened by such failures of what is otherwise expected as a matter of course. Human rights, then, can be said to be actual either as expectations or claims on the relations that are moral requisites of our individual and communal life.

---

children, is sexual fidelity within the marital relation. The use of the term "moral" is something I have discussed extensively in *Rethinking Rights and Responsibilities* in chaps. 7–9.

Human rights are inalienable. They are rendered actual as expectations of, or claims upon, a continuous set of morally significant relations, created and sustained by proclivities and inhibitions that continue to fuel these relations. Consider the simple fact that each of us is the offspring of parents. We owe them our lives. We also owe our lives to the larger community in which their behavior and our lives were sustained and protected. What we owe was made possible by the morally responsible behavior, the morally significant relations, I have identified as the moral requisites of individual and communal life. In turn, all of those who have sustained our lives, and still do, expect from us and stand ready to claim from us behavior that is in accord with the moral requisites of individual and communal life. We cannot, by wishing it to be so, divest ourselves of these responsibilities and the rights they render actual. They belong to us and to all of us as individuals and members of communities. They are inalienable.

Now consider what is implied by this account of the inalienability of the right to life. Ronald Dworkin and five other moral philosophers submitted an amicus curiae brief to the Supreme Court in support of an individual right to PAS.[19] In this brief, they recognized that the state has interests that justify limiting the right to PAS. They suggested that the state could deny some requests for PAS. The state could do so out of concern for those people who are not terminally ill but who have nevertheless formed a desire to die. The reason the state could legitimate denying PAS to this group of persons is that they "are, as a group, very likely later to be grateful if they are prevented from taking their own lives."[20] These authors are making gratitude for one's life contingent upon whether or not people actually feel it. This is not surprising given the fact that their basis for favoring a right to PAS is that the Supreme Court should recognize that an individual has a right to live or die on the basis of "his own convictions about why his life is valuable and where its value lies."[21] Dworkin et alia have provided us no basis for saying that each of us *ought* to be grateful for our lives. Our lives did not and could not originate and persist because we valued it but because someone else valued it, parents to begin with, but also a whole

---

19. "Brief of Ronald Dworkin et al.," 183–98.
20. Ibid., 196.
21. Ibid., 197.

network of individuals and groups. Our lives depended upon and continue to depend on the persistence of the moral behavior that makes life, and the communal protection of it, possible at all. This behavior is expected and claimed as a right by all. What we owe then is to behave in these same ways. Whether in living in accord with the moral responsibilities that initiate and sustain individuals and communal life we feel gratitude or not, we are doing what a grateful individual would do, namely, doing unto others as they have done unto us. This we ought to do. And to do it out of gratitude would be virtuous and would strengthen the proclivities and inhibitions to act as we ought. What we owe one another are responsibilities that remain, whether we live up to them or not. They are the inalienable natural bases of our rights. Being terminally ill does not change this reality.

But is it not the case that, despite the continuities exhibited by the proclivities and inhibitions that actualize the moral requisites of individual and communal life, individuals and groups violate or break with these continuously binding moral responsibilities humans have toward one another? There is no question that individuals and groups sometimes act in ways that run counter to their moral responsibilities.[22] That is why it is universally deemed necessary to have laws, law enforcement agencies, and military forces, in order to try to prevent killing and even threats to assault or kill human beings. Were I deliberately to kill an innocent person, that is, kill an individual who is not threatening me in any way, I would be breaking with the relation of mutual responsibilities that we share, the mutual responsibilities to protect human life. In doing this, I would have overcome my inhibitions against killing in such a way that I would be rightly seen as a threat to all other human beings. I would also correctly be seen as a threat to the inhibitions against killing present in my larger community, particularly those of individuals, families, or other groups who had great affection for the victim.

---

22. Someone like Reinhold Niebuhr would state the matter much more strongly. Niebuhr finds that all our actions less than fully meet our moral responsibilities. "Equal justice," he says, "is the approximation of brotherhood under conditions of sin." *The Nature and Destiny of Man II* (New York: Scribner's Sons, 1964), 254. Indeed, in *Moral Man and Immoral Society* (New York: Charles Scribner's Sons, 1932), Niebuhr argued that actions carried out by groups were always tainted by the biases and loyalties of those belonging to the groups in question. In short, human beings fall short of meeting their moral responsibilities; they do so imperfectly; acting as nations or on behalf of nations, they are capable of great evil, as in World War II.

In short, I would be a threat to others and to the moral fabric of my community. To deal with this, my larger community would act to try to neutralize and ward off these threats by depriving me of my usual rights to freedom. What would be done depends upon the procedures and policies in place in a community, ranging from imprisonment to capital punishment. Societies vary in the ways they deal with homicide. But, apart from exceptions such as unavoidable accidents and self-defense, killing individuals evokes responses, through laws and enforcement agencies, that attempt to neutralize or otherwise remove any threat to others and to the moral requisites of individual and communal life that any individual or group may pose were they to kill and remain free and unpunished.

What about killing oneself? In this instance as well the moral responsibilities to protect human life are violated and the inhibitions of others against killing are threatened. Indeed, we know as a matter of fact that there are copycat suicides as well as murders. Highly publicized suicides are almost invariably followed by other suicides. The moral responsibility to prevent the death of individuals, innocent of any crime, is, as noted above, continuous. Committing suicide is a failure in such a moral responsibility. The policy in place in the United States undoubtedly does not call for punishing anyone in the event of an unassisted suicide. That is justifiable. For one thing, any punishment of the victim would adversely affect only those who had close ties with that individual and, if they did not assist in or encourage that individual to commit suicide, they in no way, relative to this event, have done anything to threaten others or the moral fabric. Secondly, it is always possible that the individuals committing suicide cannot be held morally responsible for what they did because they were clinically depressed. There is no fair way to judge them. However, those who advocate PAS are urging that suicide can be rational, and hence those who commit it can be held morally responsible for what they do. Those who see themselves as rationally and intentionally justified in killing themselves are intending to act in a way that violates and threatens our mutual moral responsibilities to one another. Furthermore, they are encouraging such actions.

What about those who willingly assist in a suicide? They are willing accomplices in behavior that violates and threatens the moral fabric of our communities in the ways depicted above. What is more, their willingness to assist is an encouragement to someone seriously contemplating suicide. At the time of a study of hospice patients in England, none of the patients who had AIDS and asked to have their lives ended actually persisted in their requests.[23] In the Netherlands, under the care of physicians willing to assist AIDS patients to end their lives and legally permitted to do so, euthanasia was administered in 30 percent of the cases.[24] What happens in the Netherlands illustrates both the influence of physicians on patients and the influence of laws on both. Law does have a pedagogical effect on behavior.[25] Furthermore, the inhibitions of medical professionals against killing have been weakened in the Netherlands. Witness the documented instances of involuntary euthanasia and the reasons given for carrying them out, despite the legal criteria forbidding euthanasia without informed consent.[26]

Killing, then, is wrong when it is wrong because the act of killing oneself or someone else violates and threatens to undermine the mutual moral responsibilities that are requisites of individual and communal life. In so doing it violates an individual's natural and inalienable right to life and all the expectations and claims it makes on human behavior.

But killing can be wrong for yet another reason: when it is an act that no longer exhibits a love for life. The moral structure depicted above is not recognized as such by those who do not judge what is moral from the standpoint of wishing the self and the other to exist. Rehnquist, in discussing the wrongfulness of killing oneself, called attention to the idea, expressed by a jurist in the past, that the love of life acts to keep suicide a relatively rare phenomenon. What is the role of "love of life" in morality? That is the question we will now address.

The Love of Life. On the love of life, Rehnquist cited Zephaniah Swift, the legal theorist who became Chief Justice of Connecticut. Having argued the case for abolishing punishment for suicide, Swift

---

23. Reported in Twycross, "Where there is hope, there is life: a view from the hospice," 152–54.

24. Ibid.

25. Mary Ann Glendon discusses the law as a teacher in *Rights Talk: The Impoverishment of Political Discourse* (New York: Free Press, 1991), 85–88, including a study of how law guides one's conduct and opinions.

26. See Carlos Gomez, *Regulating Death: Euthanasia and the Case of the Netherlands* (New York: Free Press, 1991); Herbert Hendin, *Seduced by Death: Doctors, Patients, and the Dutch Cure* (New York: W. W. Norton, 1997). Hendin's work has many further references. See also footnote 68 in chap. 1 of that book.

indicated why he thought that such a change in the law would not be harmful to society. Suicide, he wrote, "is so abhorrent to the feelings of mankind, and that strong love of life which is implanted in the human heart, that it cannot be so frequently committed, as to become dangerous to society."[27] Rehnquist made the comment that Swift's statement clearly indicates that the unwillingness to punish suicide did not constitute an acceptance of suicide. Subsequent court opinions, and Rehnquist provided some examples, repudiated suicide as commendable and as a right.[28]

What is the moral significance of viewing killing oneself, and killing as such, as acts that are contrary to, and in violation of, the love of life that is implanted in us and naturally characteristic of us as human beings? One implication of taking the view that human beings naturally love life is to consider those who lose the love for their lives as deviating from normal behavior and disturbed in some way. Indeed, being suicidal became one of the major criteria for considering an individual as clinically depressed. Rehnquist took note of the high degree to which those who commit suicide had a major psychiatric illness at the time of death (his source for this puts the figure at more than 95 percent). He noted also that experiencing pain can lead to depression, and that those who are treated for depression and relieved of pain are then "grateful to be alive."[29] From a moral standpoint, attributing mental stress or illness to those who commit suicide alleviates them of any moral responsibility for killing themselves; they were not rational when they committed suicide. Furthermore, the loss of love for one's life is something that individuals and societies should always seek to correct; to do so successfully is to remove some sources of emotional or mental distress.

But apart from the extent to which the loss of love for one's life may or may not be associated with mental illness, losing love for one's life does impair moral cognition. Aristotle identified this relationship between loving one's own life and moral knowledge in his account of what it means to be a friend. To begin with, he noted that friendly relations between neighbors as well as the defining characteristics of friendships are known and attainable because of

27. *Washington v. Glucksberg*, 2264.
28. Ibid.
29. Ibid., 2272–73.

the relationships individuals have to themselves. The good we wish and do for ourselves is what we wish and do for our friends. One of the good things we wish for ourselves is to exist and live. That wish is one of the qualities that defines what it means to be a friend: "one who wishes his friend to exist and live, for his sake; which mothers do to their children."[30] This relationship of wishing oneself and another to live is a form of love, for as Aristotle says of love, it is "ideally an excess of friendship."[31] Those who love their own lives, then, know how to behave towards a neighbor and a friend; they know what it is to be a friend.

By invoking the love of mothers for their children, Aristotle is equating the love individuals have for their own lives with the natural proclivities that fuel procreation, nurture, and the wishes parents have that their children live and more.[32] Love for oneself and others, expressed in wishing oneself and others to exist, is, then, for Aristotle a natural expression of love, like that of being a parent. However, these natural expressions of love can be weakened or undermined. One source for this, as Aristotle describes it, is that people can be at variance with themselves as they follow their own desires:

> This is true, for instance, of incontinent people; for they choose instead of the things they themselves think good, things that are pleasant but hurtful; while others again, through cowardice and laziness, shrink from doing what they think best for themselves.[33]

And individuals "who have done many terrible deeds and are hated for their wickedness even shrink from life and destroy themselves."[34] So, for Aristotle, the diminution or extinction of the love of one's life is not only possible, but may even result in the destruction of one's own life. For, as Aristotle observes of wicked people, "having nothing loveable in them, they have no feeling of love to them-

---

30. Aristotle, *Nichomachean Ethics,* Book IX, Chap. 4.
31. Ibid., Book IX, Chap. 10.
32. In a transcultural study, the psychologist Tamara Dembo found that parents and future parents commonly wish "health," "economic security," "knowledge" or "intelligence," and "happy marriage" (or "loving" or "being loved"). Reported in Charles Reynolds, "Elements of a Decision Procedure for Christian Social Ethics," *Harvard Theological Review* 65, no. 4 (October 1972): 513–14.
33. Aristotle, *Nicomachean Ethics,* Book IX, Chap. 4.
34. Ibid.

selves. "[35] Such individuals, then, lack the attributes needed to know how to be a friend or be moved to be one; they will also lack the attributes characteristic of mutual parental love and the understanding of what it takes to be a loving parent.

The diminution or loss of love for oneself and for one's life distorts moral cognition. Our knowledge of how we ought to behave towards others is very much dependent on knowing what is morally right behavior toward ourselves: it is wrong for you to kill or try to kill me, and hence I have a basis for thinking it would be wrong to kill or try to kill you. But if I do not wish myself to exist I may not perceive the fact that others do wish to live. Not wishing to exist, I may not regard it as wrong to be killed or to kill myself. But then I may also not regard it as wrong to kill you or to assist you to kill yourself. Since I do not wish myself to exist, I may well assume that you also do not wish to exist, even if you do not express such a wish. Furthermore, I may tend to misperceive the wishes of those who say they do not wish to live. They may be speaking out of their pain or mental distress, or they may be seeking affirmation of their lives as worthy of existence, but in the absence of a wish that I exist, I may not recognize a contrary wish in others. Indeed, I may even think that people who wish to live under certain circumstances are irrational; lacking a wish that I exist, I do not expect others to wish to live in circumstances that I regard as much worse than anything I am experiencing.

Someone might object at this point to this line of reasoning. What would be wrong, they might contend, with wishing myself to exist but imagining that I and anyone else might understandably lose that wish under very dire circumstances when dying and near death? One can grant that such a loss of the wish to live is not only understandable but does indeed occur, though temporarily, for the great majority who are successfully treated for pain and/or clinical depression, a point discussed and documented previously. However, as I argued in the section above, our inalienable right to life rests upon our continuous and natural moral responsibilities to nurture and protect our lives. The wish no longer to assume this responsibility is a failure, either in our willingness or our emotional or mental capacity to meet that responsibility. The argument I am now putting forward is that the failure to meet that moral responsibility, whether

---

35. Ibid.

intentionally or in circumstances beyond our control, does distort our perceptions of reality, and hence also our ability to know what is right. For those who are dying, such cognitive distortions can be corrected. Obviously such changes from wishing to die to wishing to live, as the perspective from which to make moral decisions, can occur only if the efforts to bring about such changes are seen as right and are actually undertaken.

Aristotle, as quoted above, observed that people who have done many evil things will find nothing loveable in themselves and hence will not have feelings of love toward themselves. But this phenomenon obtains not only for those who have a history of doing evil, but tragically it occurs also for those who are dying, particularly those in a state of great or even complete dependence upon care from others. Individuals, highly or completely dependent on others, can come to view themselves as not at all loveable anymore. Indeed, the question of how one will be remembered, whether as vibrant, active, and attractive or as relatively helpless, debilitated, and unattractive, is among the reasons some give for wishing to end one's life either to ward off or cut short a progressive process of physical and/or mental deterioration.[36] In addition, then, to the best of care in treating pain, depression, and fear of death, it is important to address what purpose is served by dying persons who do not request PAS or euthanasia. Simply stated, such individuals fulfill some very important moral responsibilities. First of all, they do not repudiate the worth of their lives or anyone else's. Secondly, they show no ingratitude to those who brought them into being and nurtured them, those who help protect their lives, and those who have so far sustained their lives through all of their illnesses. Thirdly, they encourage no one to overcome their inhibitions against killing themselves, assisting others to do so, or killing others. Fourthly, they directly encourage those who are experiencing illnesses that may only temporarily or partially render them quite helpless, or disfigured, or dependent on others, to persist in that state and sustain their hope that the love for their lives will be sustained and may grow. Fifthly, as studies have shown, they create opportunities for spiritual growth, the deepening of existing relationships, and, in some cases, the healing of ruptured relations whether with other persons or the Divine.

---

36. *Compassion in Dying v. State of Washington* (1996), 814.

These same moral responsibilities and spiritual opportunities that characterize patients who do not request PAS or euthanasia also characterize physicians who do not practice PAS and euthanasia. These patients and physicians help sustain the moral requisites of individual and communal life and the natural proclivities and inhibitions that structure and uphold our common moral life in this way. By refraining from participation in PAS and euthanasia, physicians and patients, and other potential participants, are refusing to violate the sacredness of human life. Violating the sacredness of human life is a third reason Rehnquist gave for the wrongness of killing when it is wrong.

The Sacredness of Human Life. As indicated in chapter 2, Rehnquist called attention to the significance in law of the sacredness of human life. He cited the Model Penal Code of 1980. That code asserts that "the interests in the sanctity of life are represented in the criminal homicide laws" and are "threatened" by anyone "who expresses a willingness to participate in taking the life of another, even though the act may be accomplished with the consent, or at the request, of the suicide victim."[37] That an individual's life is sacred is continuous and in no way contingent upon life's circumstances: the right to life is both "inalienable" and "sacred."[38] These affirmations are explicitly found in court decisions. Granted, then, that violating and even threatening to undermine the sacredness of human life serves as a standard in law for judging the wrongness of killing and assisting in a suicide, is there a moral justification for its use as a reason to consider the taking of human life as morally and legally wrong when it is wrong?

As a standard for judging behavior, sacredness of life is a particular way of characterizing the worth of human life. That a human life is sacred means that the worth of it is beyond calculation, that is, incalculable. One can glean this from what is said about the sanctity of life in the citations provided by Rehnquist. An individual's life is to be protected in every imaginable circumstance: as a prisoner on death row; as hopelessly ill or fatally wounded; and as one for whom life has in various ways become a burden.[39] In other words,

---

37. *Washington v. Glucksberg*, 2265.
38. Ibid.
39. Ibid. The philosopher Frances M. Kamm has argued with great care and clarity that there are circumstances in which "death is the lesser evil" relative to continuing to live; see "Physician-Assisted Suicide, Euthanasia, and Intending Death," in

the law's interest in preserving life is unqualified. This interest is not diminished in any way by the medical condition and the wishes of the one whose life is at stake. Washington State rejects any sliding scale that would seek to calculate the degree of interest the state should take in an individual's life. Rehnquist affirmed the right of states to refrain from making judgments about the quality of life that a particular individual may enjoy.[40]

As embodied in law, the sacredness of life refers to the incalculable worth of life. In the German Constitutional Court, the judges recognized the necessity of embedding in law the incalculable worth of individual human life. The Weimer Constitution had made no explicit reference to the right to life. Mindful of all that happened during the period of the Nazi regime, the Basic Law of what was then West Germany incorporated "the self-evident right to life" and did so "principally as a reaction to the destruction of life unworthy of life."[41] Dr. Benda, writing for the court, made this same point in yet another way. Speaking of the Basic Law, he asserted that

---

Physician-Assisted Suicide: Expanding the Debate, ed. Margaret P. Battin et al. (New York: Routledge, 1998), 28–62. This argument, if accepted, would remove the current protection of life in homicide law that is not contingent upon any of the circumstances Kamm suggests; Kamm does not consider what principle guides, or even should guide, homicide law; she also does not consider how acts of suicide, assisting in them, and the practice of euthanasia affect the inhibitions and proclivities essential to the moral requisites of individual and communal life and essential for the enforcement of homicide law. She has totally individualized the calculus of whether it is best to die rather than live with virtually no regard to the ways in which individuals are related to one another.

40. *Washington v. Glucksberg,* 2272. When I speak of life's worth as incalculable, I am, of course refraining from making judgments about life's worth based on any assessment of anyone's quality of life. In the past, I opposed such quality of life judgments by asserting that all life is of equal worth. To me, that meant: (1) that no one's life is worth more than that of another; and (2) that no one's life can or should be considered of any more or less worth, whatever its circumstances or condition. Nancy Platteborze, currently studying with me as a doctoral student in ethics at Harvard, pointed out, quite rightly, that what I was trying to express is that life's worth is beyond calculation. It is confusing to use a term like "equal" since it conjures up the idea of numerical comparisons, precisely what I was seeking to avoid. I am most grateful for her discernment and assistance. As the reader will note, I have, throughout this book, represented my view of life's worth by speaking of the *incalculable worth of life,* of life's worth as *beyond calculation.*

41. This is in the decision of the Federal Constitutional Court of West Germany, published in full as "West German Abortion Decision: A Contrast to Roe v. Wade?" Robert E. Jonas and John D. Gorby, trans., *John Marshall Journal of Practice and Procedure* 9 (Spring 1976): 605–84. Page references to this decision are to the reprint in S. J. Reiser, A. J. Dyck, and W. J. Curran, eds., *Ethics in Medicine* (Cambridge: MIT Press, 1977), 417.

at its basis lies the concept...that human beings possess an inherent worth as individuals in order of creation which uncompromisingly demands unconditional respect for the life of every individual human being, even for the apparently socially "worthless...."[42]

What makes killing morally wrong, then, when it is wrong, is that a human life, the one killed, is treated as a life that has little or no worth rather than as a life of incalculable worth and as one having a right to be treated accordingly. If laws were permitted to embody the idea that in some circumstances life loses its worth, or that some people lack sufficient worth to have their lives protected, individuals would no longer enjoy equal protection of the law so far as their lives are concerned. Furthermore, some principled basis for protecting human life other than its sanctity would have to be provided to justify what would constitute violations of the unquestioned worth of every individual human life.

Ronald Dworkin has proposed legalizing PAS because, in doing so, the law would recognize the sacredness of individual human life, not violate it. The basis for his argument is that whether or not the sacredness of life requires death due to natural causes or death at a time of one's choosing is a matter of religious belief. People have different beliefs about how their lives should end and what their choices mean. The law should be neutral with regard to these beliefs and should not suppress individual religious beliefs, particularly in such a personal and important matter about which beliefs differ. He makes this point rather strongly when he states that "making someone die in a way that others approve," but the individual whose life it is "believes" to be "a horrifying contradiction of his life, is a devastating, odious form of tyranny."[43] That is a rather passionate rejection of what the Supreme Court decided. In fact, as the reader will recall, Dworkin joined five other philosophers in urging the Supreme Court, as it was deciding the question, to recognize PAS as a constitutional right.[44] In what sense, then, is human life sacred for Dworkin? "Something is sacred or inviolable," Dworkin tells us, "when its deliberate destruction would dishonor what ought to

---

42. Ibid., 424.
43. Ronald Dworkin, *Life's Dominion: An Argument about Abortion, Euthanasia, and Individual Freedom* (New York: Vintage Books, 1994), 217.
44. "Brief of Ronald Dworkin et al."

be honored."[45] Dworkin uses the terms "sacred" and "inviolable" as synonyms. By this definition, how could the deliberate ending of a human life be compatible with its sacredness? Dworkin develops the notion that each individual life represents a whole way of life. Our lives tell a story about us and how that story ends is very important to us, like the final scene in a drama. For most people, Dworkin contends, how they die has "special, symbolic importance: they want their deaths, if possible, to express and in that way vividly to confirm the values they believe most important in their lives."[46] Timing has this kind of significance for "the idea of a good (or less bad) death."[47] In short, Dworkin claims: "None of us wants to end our lives out of character."[48] For some, dying at the time and in the manner that they choose is the way to respect the inviolability of human life.[49] People's lives differ, and so do their beliefs as to how their own lives should end. Each person's belief about what it means to treat one's own life as sacred is a personal belief. Dworkin regards that belief as a religious belief. The law should not suppress such religious beliefs because to do so violates the sacredness of life as some individuals understand its meaning. These are individuals who believe it is intolerable, utterly undignified, to live under some circumstances that severely limit their physical or mental abilities. Dworkin summarizes his views as follows:

> Because we cherish dignity, we insist on freedom, and we place the right of conscience at its center, so that a government that denies that right is totalitarian no matter how free it leaves us in choices that matter less. Because we have dignity, we demand democracy, and we define it so that a constitution that permits a majority to deny freedom of conscience is democracy's enemy, not its author. Whatever view we take about . . . euthanasia, we want the right to decide for ourselves, and we should therefore be ready to insist that any honorable constitution, any genuine constitution of principle, will guarantee that right for everyone.[50]

---

45. Ronald Dworkin, *Life's Dominion*, 74.
46. Ibid., 211. This concern with what one's death expresses includes the concern about how one is remembered, 210.
47. Ibid.
48. Ibid., 213.
49. Ibid., 216.
50. Ibid., 239.

In this passage, Dworkin equates a total ban on euthanasia with a totalitarian denial of freedom of conscience. But he is begging the question. The question is about practices that should or should not be permitted by law. First I would distinguish between a religious belief and the actions or practices favored by that belief. There have been, and still are, people whose religious beliefs incline them to favor polygamy. However, the Supreme Court and the laws of the land do not legally permit the practice of that belief.[51] Holding the belief is certainly legally permitted. I do not know whether Dworkin agrees with the Supreme Court decisions to which the preceding footnote refers, but they illustrated the distinction between beliefs and practices as recognized in law. It would be one thing to believe in child sacrifice; it would be quite another to practice it. I do not expect that Dworkin, however tolerant of another's religious beliefs, would wish to have such a practice legally permitted. People, as Dworkin knows, are not free to follow their consciences when it comes to killing others or helping others kill themselves. We have abolished such practices as dueling, for example, a practice in which people defended their honor or dignity. Nor can people avenge a wrong they have suffered even when they rightly see their cause as just. Rather, as a society, we say we believe in the rule of law in such matters.

And so the question before us is whether we also accept the rule of law when it comes to PAS and euthanasia, or whether we think it is a matter for individual consciences, rather than the common morality as now embedded in law.

As we noted earlier, the American Bar Association, in its Model Penal Code of 1980, took the view that the sanctity or sacredness of human life is threatened by those who would willingly participate in any act that would take the life of another individual, even if the individual who commits suicide requests that participation. How is such a threat best understood? As indicated earlier as well, in current law a human life is sacred in the sense that its worth is incalculable and the interest of the State in protecting it unqualified. Furthermore, the love of life is a natural phenomenon. Human beings who procreate, nurture, and protect one another are expressing

---

51. Polygamy and the relevant Supreme Court decisions regarding this practice are discussed in Mary Ann Glendon, *The Transformation of Family Law: State, Law, and Family in the United States and Western Europe* (Chicago: University of Chicago Press, 1989), 52–55.

such a love for life. But life is also protected by the strong inhibitions against killing and being killed. It would be extremely difficult to enforce the laws against homicide if human beings had no inhibitions against killing and/or were inclined to hate life, their own and that of others.

Having just laws and order in a community is extremely important. In a situation in which law and order has broken down, individuals who have some hatreds or are seeking revenge may well overcome their usual inhibitions against killing. Once they do, their sense of the worth of a human life, their own and that of others, may decline markedly, or even disappear. Consider the following account, gleaned in an interview of a Bosnian Serb sniper who killed Muslims in Sarajevo during the conflict there in the early years of the past decade. His name is Pipo. He claims to have killed 325 people. He tells the interviewer that he is not sure now that he is a normal person because he only knows how to kill, and he will even kill someone who is talking with him, if pushed: "In the beginning, . . . I put my fear aside. . . . Then with the killings, I put my emotions aside. . . . But now they are gone."[52]

Pipo used to run a restaurant with a Muslim as his partner. That was before the war. Pipo joined the Bosnian Serb army, but his hatred for Muslims did not begin until after his mother was jailed and beaten by them and, when released, would not speak about what happened. "That's when," says Pipo, "I picked up a gun and started shooting Muslims. I hate them all."[53] An officer in the sniper unit he joined taught him a useful mental technique to help him carry out his task: he told Pipo not to let the faces of those he shoots "follow him." Pipo learned to do his work well, but he lost all of his normal feelings, even feelings of affection for his mother, the feelings that first drove him to avenge her victimization. After he last saw his mother, Pipo says of that encounter, "She hugged me and I felt nothing. . . . I have no life anymore. . . . I don't want a wife and children."[54] As reported, the interview with Pipo concludes after Pipo sends a visitor a note and some cigarettes to take to a friend who is a Muslim sniper and was his opponent in the war.

---

52. Edward Barnes, "A Sniper's Tale," *Time* (March 19, 1994), 24.
53. Ibid.
54. Ibid.

When he is asked whether he would kill that Muslim if he got him in the sights of his gun, he simply replied, "Why not?"[55]

This is a rather graphic account of an individual who has lost the love of life and the proclivities and inhibitions that nourish and sustain it. Life has consequently no worth to him; neither his own, nor that of others. The sacredness of life has effectively no meaning for him. He calls the continuation of his life as a killer his own choice. Would Dworkin grant Pipo "freedom of conscience" for the choices he is making? I think not.

Dworkin could consider this story an extreme one, but it illustrates what can and does happen when the inhibitions against killing weaken sufficiently. In the initial government study of euthanasia as practiced in the Netherlands, physicians reported that, contrary to the legal rules governing the practice of it, they sometimes ended the lives of competent patients who had not requested euthanasia. The major reasons given were that the quality of life of these patients was very low and their families could not stand it any longer.[56] If such physicians still retained strong inhibitions against killing, they would surely have wanted their competent patients to tell them how they believed their lives should end, and whether they believed the sacredness of life could still be upheld by them were they to request and receive euthanasia or assisted suicide.

Even the inhibition against killing animals, particularly pets, can be weakened. A veterinarian confided in me that she had had a difficult struggle, emotionally, when she first gave a lethal injection to a dog under her care even though it had the consent of the owners and it seemed to her a merciful thing to do. But, after administering euthanasia to a number of pet animals in the course of her practice, she had a shocking thought one day: she was killing these animals without any of the hesitations and emotional regrets she had felt when she did it for the first time.[57]

What I have been arguing is that "the sacredness of life" is a term that describes the worth of all individual human life as incalculable. Human beings naturally have the proclivities and inhibitions that sustain this idea of life's worth and the love for it. The laws against homicide are an expression of the community's interest, through its

---

55. Ibid.

56. See R. Fenigsen, "The Report of the Dutch Governmental Committee on Euthanasia," *Issues in Law and Medicine* 7, no. 3 (Winter 1991): 343.

57. Lisa Fullam, personal communication.

laws, to maintain the proclivities and inhibitions that render it at all possible to retain the sacredness of life as a standard of conduct and as a reality of communal life. After all, nurturing and protecting life are moral requisites of individual and communal life. Permitting in law the willingness to ask others to kill oneself, and the willingness to honor such a request, directly sanctions acts and practices that overcome the inhibitions against killing and the proclivity to nurture life, in oneself and others. To qualify what it means to call life sacred is to qualify or render contingent the incalculable worth of each individual life. If the law permits people to act on the premise that a life may not be worth living, by what moral principle and by what law does one prevent suicide and homicide? By what moral principle does one say that any deeply held wish to kill or be killed is a violation of the sacredness of human life that is the standard for protecting all individual human lives?

Dworkin would reply that it is possible to limit the freedom to kill and to assist in a suicide. Recognizing a need to limit assisted suicide, Dworkin, along with five other moral philosophers, suggested the following:

> A state might assert, for example, that people who are not terminally ill, but who have formed a desire to die, are, as a group, very likely later to be grateful if they are prevented from taking their own lives. It might then be legitimate, out of concern for such people, to deny them a doctor's assistance.[58]

Interestingly enough, this proposal, indirectly at least, acknowledges a general love of life and the desirability of retaining some support for it in law. At the same time, it is a departure from the strict association of dignity with the individual's own convictions in matters of when and how to die. It directly contradicts one of Dworkin's dicta, namely: "Value cannot be poured into a life from the outside; it must be generated by the person whose life it is."[59] To assume that all people will be grateful to be denied assistance in ending their lives, provided they are not terminally ill, is to value their lives from the outside, unless one also assumes that individuals naturally, or otherwise, love their own lives. If that is being assumed by Dworkin, then he is claiming that terminal illness can be expected

58. "Brief of Ronald Dworkin et al.," 196.
59. Dworkin, *Life's Dominion*, 230.

to undermine the love of life and render life unworthy of life, at least for some people. But only when caregivers and lawgivers act on the assumption that the terminally ill will be grateful for life once they are properly cared for does the opportunity for that gratitude emerge for those who had been expressing a wish to die.

Dr. Herbert Hendin, an American psychiatrist, has called attention to the powerful influence of physicians in the decisions of patients who are gravely or terminally ill.[60] In his analysis of the case of Diane, he noted the ways in which Dr. Timothy Quill, whose views were cited in chapter 2, aided his patient not only to carry out her death by suicide, but also influenced her to make that very decision.[61] Hendin contends that Quill and other physicians tend to overlook and fail to treat their patients' fear of death. To illustrate how this can change the outlook of patients and focus a patient on whatever life may still offer, he presented a case of a patient with Diane's same disease:

> Like Diane, Tim was given a 25 percent chance of survival. His immediate reaction was a desperate preoccupation with suicide and a wish for support in carrying it out. At first he could not consider how he felt about death and its meaning to him but remained preoccupied with concerns about being dependent and unwilling to tolerate the symptoms of his disease or the side effects of proposed treatment. Once we could talk about the possibility of his dying—what it meant to him in terms of separation and bodily disintegration—his desperate avoidance subsided. He decided to undergo medical treatment, complained relatively little about the unpleasant side effects, and used the remaining months of his life to connect with his wife and parents in ways that were meaningful for him. Two days before he died, Tim talked of what he would have missed without the opportunity for a loving parting.[62]

---

60. Herbert Hendin, "Seduced by Death: Doctors, Patients, and the Dutch Cure," *Issues in Law and Medicine* 10, no. 2 (Fall 1994): 123–68.

61. Ibid., 125–28. For the case of Diane, see Timothy Quill, "Death and Dignity: A Case of Individualized Decision-Making," *New England Journal of Medicine* 324, no. 10 (March 7, 1991): 691–94. See also Stephanie Jamison, *Assisted Suicide: A Decision-Making Guide for Health Professionals* (San Francisco: Jossey-Bass Publishers, 1998).

62. Hendin, "Seduced by Death," 128.

Under the care of someone like Dr. Hendin, patients like Tim have the opportunity to affirm their lives and find meaning in life, while knowing full well that they are dying. Reacting to the considerable data on the practice of euthanasia in the Netherlands, Hendin has concluded: "Euthanasia, fought for on the basis of the principle of autonomy and self-determination of patients, has actually increased the paternalistic power of the medical profession."[63] Most Dutch physicians oppose the legislation that requires them to report cases in which patient's lives have been ended without their express wishes or consent. Why should they be expected to turn themselves in for a crime? One such physician, Dr. Herbert Cohen, is quoted by Dr. Hendin as saying, "Death is influenced by a doctor's decision in almost all nontraumatic cases. Death is an orchestrated happening."[64] That the doctor is "the conductor of the orchestra" has aroused concern among even the most avid supporters of assisted suicide and euthanasia: they are becoming aware of too many physicians who are unaware of how the moods and wishes of patients can fluctuate, moods and wishes that can change during the course of treatment.[65]

The influence over how patients view their lives and whether they decide to end them does not stop with terminally ill patients. Patients who are not terminally ill can be persuaded to view their illness in such a way that they react to it as though it were a terminal illness or, in any event, an illness they should consider intolerable. Dr. Richard Fenigsen, long a medical practitioner in the Netherlands, has reported just such a case.[66] The patient, Mrs. P., was a seventy-two-year-old widow with a heart condition that responded well to treatment. She was living independently, though she needed help to keep her house clean and her exercise was limited to walking a few blocks. She did sometimes come in with symptoms, but they were successfully dealt with. Dr. Fenigsen described Mrs. P. as "an extremely nice, mild-tempered lady who never showed any impatience and complied with the doctor's every order and advice."[67] When Mrs. P. failed to appear at the outpatient clinic as expected,

---

63. Ibid., 163.
64. Ibid., 160.
65. Ibid.
66. Richard Fenigsen, "Physician-Assisted Death in the Netherlands: Impact on Long-Term Care," *Issues in Law and Medicine* 11, no. 3 (Winter 1995): 283–97.
67. Ibid., 295.

Dr. Fenigsen contacted her family physician. This is what he told Dr. Fenigsen he had done:

> He had a talk with Mrs. P.... and explained the situation to her: This wasn't going to be any better, and living such a limited life, with all those pills, made no sense at all. Mrs. P. accepted everything he said, he stopped her pills, and three days later she died.[68]

Fenigsen said that he was overcome by deep sorrow and that it returns every time he thinks of Mrs. P. She could have lived considerably longer.

Fenigsen assures the reader that this is not an isolated case of physicians convincing patients that they should die and then acting to end their lives. He cited the following data published by the Dutch Government Committee on Euthanasia:

> In 1990 about 86,000 people died while under medical care, and in 49,000 of these cases (57 percent) doctors at some point made decisions that could, or did, hasten deaths. In 14,550 cases the (medically not futile) life-prolonging treatment was withdrawn or withheld with intention to terminate life. Sixty-five percent of family physicians believe that doctors may propose (active) euthanasia to a patient who does not ask for it himself.[69]

From these cases and these data, we can observe that the beliefs of physicians regarding the sacredness of human life can influence and even shape the beliefs and actions of their patients. However intimate and personal end of life decisions may be, what these will be is much more dependent upon what others, particularly physicians, believe than Dworkin acknowledges. Dworkin unrealistically depicts individuals as quite disconnected from others with respect to what meaning and worth they give to their lives. What whole communities, loved ones, and physicians believe about the sacredness of individual human life has much more significance for each of us as individuals than Dworkin leads us to believe.

From these cases and these data we can also observe that what the law has to say about the sacredness of life also influences and shapes

---

68. Ibid.
69. Ibid.

the beliefs of patients and physicians. A complete ban on assisted suicide embodies in law the core of what it means to call life sacred; individual human life retains its incalculable worth in all circumstances. It gives every individual and health professional a moral and legal reason to try to prevent suicide, as well as to alleviate any mental and/or physical distress that may tempt or drive someone to do it. However, if physicians and patients are legally permitted actively to kill, kill themselves, or assist others to kill themselves, some individuals, whether freely or under someone else's influence, will not have the opportunity to have their love of life sustained and supported in a way that inspires gratitude. And it was the potential for gratitude that Dworkin and his associates claimed should allow the states to deny physician assistance in a suicide. I agree that this is a reason for denying PAS, but I disagree that it applies only to individuals who are not terminally ill. It is a reason to deny PAS to everyone. As I argued, people ought to be grateful for life and ought to act in ways that help support the proclivities and inhibitions that sustain individual and communal life. And Dworkin does not give us any reason to believe that people will be grateful when they are prevented from committing suicide. He has implied but not affirmed that people do have a natural love of life, a love which, as I have indicated, expresses itself in the procreation, nurture, and protection of human life. This love is strong enough to yield an ever-growing number of people on this earth, despite all of the deaths that result from wars and natural disasters.

With regard to the consequences of permitting physicians to assist in suicide, Dworkin focuses exclusively on freedom of conscience for patients. We have already noted that this is a much more limited freedom than Dworkin hypothesizes. And, of course, ending one's life is the ultimate in destroying any freedom an individual may still retain while terminally or seriously ill. But Dworkin ignores what happens to physicians. They are free to follow their consciences on what they think is a life worth living and free to influence people to act on the physicians' beliefs, as we have noted. Furthermore, the physicians themselves are partly, perhaps very strongly, swayed by what the law teaches them. This would appear to be the case in the Netherlands. Fenigsen is convinced that the growing preference for assisted suicide and euthanasia, even without requests for them, has mostly come after the courts there permitted physicians to honor requests for ending lives using lethal means. He experienced that among his medical colleagues, and the data support his reflection.[70]

Dworkin has dismissed appeals to what has been happening in the Netherlands, although I have difficulty with that view. However, more importantly, Dworkin has not provided a moral justification for preventing suicide, other than his appeal to gratitude: he has not, as I argued above, given us a reason to expect gratitude for having our lives saved. He does not explicitly affirm the natural love for life that would lead us to expect such gratitude.

Dworkin and his associates reject any suggestion of a slippery slope. But the German Constitutional Court responded self-consciously to the very idea that there is such a thing as a "life unworthy of life." They knew what actions accord with the belief that life is something less than an ultimate, incalculable value. Mindful also that the law is a teacher, the Court had this to say about how human life should be valued. Noting that Germany's Basic Law guarantees the protection of human dignity, the Court asserted:

> Where human life exists, human dignity is present to it; it is not decisive that the bearer of this dignity himself be conscious of it and know personally how to preserve it.
>
> ... Human life represents within the order of the Basic Law, an ultimate value, the particulars of which need not be established; it is the living foundation of human dignity and the prerequisite for all other fundamental rights.[71]

These passages are a clear expression of the inviolability of life and of its incalculable worth: they comport with what I think it means to refer to life as sacred. And protecting human life, on this view, is at once a protection of human dignity at its core and of all other rights, including individual freedom. Permitting PAS and euthanasia is compromising the freedom of many patients in the Netherlands, understandably so. In one sense, the freedom of all patients is compromised by permitting physicians to offer PAS. Offering PAS is something American laws on informed consent would undoubtedly require, if PAS were to become a constitutional right.

---

70. Ibid.
71. "West German Abortion Decision," 419.

TOWARD A SYNTHESIS OF EXISTING TRADITIONS

Dworkin distinguishes between two schools of thought about how to make decisions within constitutional law: the "Party of History" and the "Party of Principle." Chief Justice Rehnquist belongs to the "Party of History"; Judge Reinhardt belongs to the "Party of Principle." Their reasoning on PAS followed the very methods and schools of thought with which Dworkin would identify them. Dworkin has expressed his clear preference for the "Party of Principle."[72]

As I have argued in chapter 3, Reinhardt is wedded to what he regards as Millian principles. But, as I argued in that chapter as well, his version of Mill does not attend to certain aspects of Mill's more comprehensive views, particularly with regard to the need for certain moral rules and with regard to the harm that would ensue if such moral rules were undermined or abolished. We now turn to consider John Stuart Mill's account of these moral rules.

Mill distinguishes two kinds of moral obligations or duties. Perfect duties are those that individuals may claim from us as a right; imperfect duties do not give rise to anything that may be claimed as a right. Justice refers to a set of perfect obligations. "Justice," Mill says, "implies something which it is not only right to do and wrong not to do, but which some individual can claim from us as his moral right."[73] In defining justice, Mill refers to this set of perfect obligations as moral rules:

> Justice is a name for certain classes of moral rules which con-
> cern the essentials of human well-being more nearly, and are
> therefore of more absolute obligation than any other rules for
> the guidance of life; and the notion which we have found to
> be of the essence of the idea of justice, that of a right resid-

---

72. This distinction is found in Ronald Dworkin, "Sex, Death and the Courts," *New York Review of Books,* August 8, 1996, 44–50. See James M. DuBois, "Physician-Assisted Suicide and Public Virtue: A Reply to the Liberty Thesis of 'The Philosopher's Brief,' " *Issues in Law and Medicine* 15, no. 2 (Fall 1999): 176–77, for a critique of Dworkin for siding with one method of interpreting the Constitution to the exclusion of the other.

73. John Stuart Mill, "Utilitarianism," in *The Philosophy of John Stuart Mill,* ed. Marshall Cohen (New York: Random House, 1961), 380. Mill uses the terms "obligations" and "duties" interchangeably.

ing in an individual, implies and testifies to this more binding obligation.[74]

Just before defining justice, Mill calls it "the chief part, and incomparably the most sacred and binding part, of all morality."[75]

Why does Mill describe the moral rules as so very sacred and binding? For one thing, they forbid human beings to hurt one another, and that is "more vital to human well-being than rules that only indicate how best to manage some of our activities."[76] In addition, Mill asserts,

> They have ... the peculiarity, that they are the main element in determining the whole of the social feelings of mankind. It is their observance which alone preserves peace among human beings: if obedience to them were not the rule, and disobedience the exception, every one would see in every one else an enemy, against whom he must be perpetually guarding himself. . . . It is by a person's observance of these, that his fitness to exist as one of the fellowship of human beings is tested and decided.[77]

And, what is more, justice involves the individual's interest in security. Security, says Mill,

> no human being can possibly do without: on it we depend for all our immunity from evil, and for the whole value of all and every good ... [it is] the claim we have on our fellow-creatures to join in making safe for us the very groundwork of our existence.[78]

Clearly, Mill is describing moral rules that laws should encourage, protect, and enforce as necessary. So much is at stake: "the very groundwork of our existence" and the sustenance of the social feelings that incline us to comply with these moral rules. Does Mill give us any clue as to how these moral rules relate to the protection and worth of individual human life? He does. After repeating his point that justice names certain moral requirements "of more

---

74. Ibid., 391.
75. Ibid.
76. Ibid., 391–92.
77. Ibid., 392.
78. Ibid., 385.

paramount obligation than any others," he gives an example of one such duty so compelling in some situations that it can override other obligations of justice: "Thus, to save a life, it may not only be allowable, but a duty, to steal, or take by force, the necessary food or medicine, or to kidnap, and compel to officiate, the only qualified medical practitioner."[79] So despite the fact that not interfering in another's freedom is one of the moral rules of justice for Mill, saving a life takes precedence. No jurist appealing to Millian principles is true to Mill who would fail to count this as not only one of Mill's principles but as one even more compelling than the very stringent obligation to refrain from interfering with someone's freedom.

Mill also affirms the importance of protecting life by means of enforcing parental nurture. Speaking of procreation, Mill calls "causing the existence of a human being one of the most responsible actions in the range of human life."[80] It is, for Mill, irresponsible to bestow life on an individual unless the individual brought into this world has some reasonable chance at a desirable existence. Mill is ready legally to enforce the moral responsibility to nurture life. In his words,

> The laws which, in many countries on the Continent, forbid marriage unless the parties can show that they have the means of supporting a family, do not exceed the powers of the State.... They are not objectionable as violations of liberty.[81]

Interestingly enough, Mill considers gratitude to be one of the requirements of justice. Unlike Dworkin and his associates, he would expect gratitude for the gift and protection of life as something individuals ought to express in their behavior. Dworkin and his associates depict gratitude for having one's life preserved as a likely empirical contingency, not as a moral obligation. Furthermore, unlike Mill, they imagine circumstances in which they neither expect, nor morally require, gratitude for care that affirms, comforts, and continues the life of an individual who is terminally ill.

From what we have revealed of Mill's thinking about justice as the most sacred moral requirement and saving human life as the most highly obligatory requirement of justice, it is not at all evident

---

79. Ibid., 397.
80. Ibid., 310.
81. Ibid., 311.

that Mill would agree to a constitutional right to PAS. Certainly there are elements in Mill's thinking that could be construed as viewing exceptions to the ban on assisted suicide as undermining, if not violating, justice, the most sacred of moral obligations and our guarantor of individual security and our very lives.

But I do not want to speculate on how Mill would decide the issues surrounding PAS and euthanasia. Rather, I wish, more modestly, to suggest that those who are concerned to make judgments based on Millian principles should do it with full knowledge of what it would mean to do so. In accord with Mill's principles of justice, jurists should ask of any proposed constitutional right not only whether a liberty interest is at stake, but also whether the very groundwork of our existence would be undermined by granting such a liberty interest; jurists should also ask whether the social feelings that support justice and, therefore, guard the security of every individual's life, would in any way be undermined by granting such a liberty. If jurists were to take these Millian principles into account, they would be asking some of the same questions being asked by jurists who wish to protect the natural right to life and the natural responsibilities required for protecting it. Mill, as I have indicated, equates the sacredness of justice with the sacredness of life. Saving life, for Mill, upholds a social obligation.

I am not advocating that jurists base their decisions on Millian principles. Rather, I am advocating that jurists refrain from that special, selective use of Mill that suppresses the traditions that affirm our natural rights and natural responsibilities. For these traditions provide a way of thinking that seeks to uphold the inalienability of the individual right to life, the love of life, and the sacredness of each individual life, the worth of which is beyond all calculations. Those who find Mill compelling need not suppress such concerns. They can find in Mill reasons to join the effort to try to assure the security of every human life insofar as laws are necessary and able to do so. Our homicide laws try to do so. The laws against assisted suicide try to do so as well.

CONCLUDING REFLECTIONS

What I have endeavored to show is that the sacredness of life and the inalienable right to life can be morally justified. When Chief Justice Rehnquist cites the patterns of laws and judicial reasoning that support a complete ban of assisted suicide, he is appealing to traditions that affirm the protection of individual life as a natural right. Natural responsibilities are affirmed within America's biblical and theological traditions; natural rights are affirmed within America's natural rights tradition, as represented by Hobbes and Locke and those who signed the Declaration of Independence. When appealing to these traditions, it is reductionistic to suggest that this is simply an appeal to history. It is that. But it is also an appeal to principles and moral concepts that have been, and still are, embedded in and enforced by current legislation and Supreme Court decisions. These moral concepts represent a longstanding and current pattern of laws and thinking that is, for Rehnquist and many other jurists, the best guide to what amounts to a virtual consensus of the nation's conscience.[82] If this consensus is to change, the Supreme Court has unanimously agreed the change should come, for the present, from legislation enacted by democratically elected representatives of the people. Rehnquist's judicial reasoning, then, includes principles. Dworkin's distinction between the Party of Principle and the Party of History is too sharply drawn.

No one should mistake what it means to draw upon biblical and Christian affirmations. Nothing in this book constitutes an appeal to authority on my part. What I have tried to do is present reasoned arguments, appropriate to a public debate, for viewpoints currently embedded in law and used by Rehnquist to defend the Supreme Court's decision regarding assisted suicide. No one need accept the traditions that helped shape those viewpoints and the moral concepts they advocate. But if my arguments are at all persuasive, they could, on rational grounds, accept the moral concepts and the laws Rehnquist has upheld. If not, I welcome reasoned criticism from my readers and anyone else. Factually based, rational debate is essential; any outlook may be partially or wholly mistaken.

I have also endeavored to show that the traditions of natural responsibilities and natural rights that have evolved into a synthesis are not incompatible with the tradition represented by John Stuart Mill. Instead of debating conflicting theological anthropologies these traditions espouse, it is possible to derive from all three traditions a very similar concept of why individual life is sacred and should in law be viewed as such. Unlike the very narrow version of

82. *Washington v. Glucksberg*, 2263.

Mill that guides Judge Reinhardt and other jurists, all individuals should be protected from laws that would totally individualize or otherwise undermine what it means to refer to life as sacred. Unlike the view held by Reinhardt and Dworkin, among others, the laws should uphold a view of sacredness such that the law reflects, teaches, and supports the incalculable worth of the life of each individual. The law should make no exceptions that would undermine or qualify this notion of the sacredness of human life.

I have argued that legalizing PAS would constitute a violation of the natural moral responsibility to treat human beings in such a way that the worth of their lives is regarded as immeasurably valuable. I have also argued that all individuals have the inalienable right to have their lives so regarded. This responsibility and this right are moral requisites of individual and communal life. These moral requisites are rendered possible by our natural proclivities to bring life into being and to nurture and protect it morally and legally. These moral requisites are rendered possible as well by our natural inhibitions against killing. Laws should help maintain, shape, and enforce these natural proclivities and inhibitions. To do this requires laws against homicide. To do this requires, as well, specific laws against assisted suicide.

Bibliography

Aristotle. *Nichomachean Ethics.*

Barnes, Edward. "A Sniper's Tale." *Time,* March 19, 1994, 24.

Battin, M. P., R. Rhodes, and A. Silver, eds. *Physician-Assisted Suicide: Expanding the Debate.* New York: Routledge, 1998.

Beauchamp, Tom, and James F. Childress. *Principles of Biomedical Ethics.* New York: Oxford University Press, 1994.

Bentham, Jeremy. "Anarchical Fallacies." In *Society, Law, and Morality.* Ed. Frederick A. Olafson. Englewood Cliffs, N.J.: Prentice-Hall, 1961.

Bopp, James Jr., and Richard E. Coleson. "Three Strikes: Is an Assisted Suicide Right Out?" *Issues in Law and Medicine* 15, no. 1 (Summer 1999): 3–86.

Bouvia v. Superior Court, 225 Cal. Rptr. 297 (Cal. App. 2 Dist. 1986).

Brock, Dan. "Death and Dying." In *Medical Ethics.* Ed. Robert M. Veatch. Boston: Jones and Bartlett Publishers, 1989.

Brophy v. New England Sinai Hospital, 497 N.E. 2nd 626 (1986).

Brown, J. H., et al. "Is It Normal for Terminally Ill Patients to Desire Death?" *American Journal of Psychiatry* 143, no. 2 (February 1986): 208–11.

The California Death with Dignity Act. California Proposition No. 16 (1992).

Cameron, Nigel. *Death without Dignity: Euthanasia in Perspective.* Edinburgh: Rutherford House Books, 1990.

Clark, Nina. *The Politics of Physician Assisted Suicide.* New York: Garland Publishing, 1997.

Cohen, Marshall, ed. *The Philosophy of John Stuart Mill.* New York: Random House, 1961.

Compassion in Dying v. State of Washington, 850 F. Supp. 1454 (W.D. Wash. 1994).

Compassion in Dying v. State of Washington, No. 94-35534, 1995 WL 94679 (9th Cir. Mar. 9, 1995).

Compassion in Dying v. State of Washington, 79 F. 3rd 790 (9th Cir. 1996).

Compassion in Dying v. State of Washington, 85 F. 3rd 1440 (9th Cir. June 12, 1996).

Condiff, David. *Euthanasia Is Not the Answer: A Hospice Physician's View.* Clifton, N.J.: Humana Press, 1992.

Cruzan v. Director, Mo. Dept. of Health, 497 U.S. 261 (1990).

Davis, David Brion. *The Problem of Slavery in Western Culture.* Ithaca, N.Y.: Cornell University Press, 1966.

DuBois, James M. "Physician-Assisted Suicide and Public Virtue: A Reply to the Liberty Thesis of 'The Philosopher's Brief.'" *Issues in Law and Medicine* 15, no. 2 (Fall 1999): 159–79.

Dworkin, Ronald. *Life's Dominion: An Argument about Abortion, Euthanasia, and Individual Freedom.* New York: Random House, 1994.

———. "Sex, Death and the Courts." *New York Review of Books,* August 8, 1996.

———. "Brief of Ronald Dworkin, Thomas Nagel, Robert T. Nozick, John Rawls, Thomas Scanlon, and Judith Jarvis Thomson as Amici Curiae in Support of Respondents." *Issues in Law and Medicine* 15, no. 2 (Fall 1999): 183–98.

Dyck, Arthur J. *Rethinking Rights and Responsibilities: The Moral Bonds of Community.* Cleveland: Pilgrim Press, 1994.

Fenigsen, Richard. "The Report of the Dutch Governmental Committee on Euthanasia." *Issues in Law and Medicine* 7, no. 3 (Winter 1991): 339–44.

———. "Physician-Assisted Death in the Netherlands: Impact on Long-Term Care." *Issues in Law and Medicine* 11, no. 3 (Winter 1995): 283–97.

Gert, Bernard, Chares M. Culver, and K. Danner Clouser. "An Alternative to Physician-Assisted Suicide: A Conceptual and Moral Analysis." In *Physician-Assisted Suicide: Expanding the Debate.* Ed. M. P. Battin, R. Rhodes, and A. Silver. New York: Routledge, 1998.

Gewirth, Alan. *Reason and Morality.* Chicago: University of Chicago Press, 1978.

———. *Human Rights: Essays on Justification and Applications.* Chicago: University of Chicago Press, 1982.

Glendon, Mary Ann. *The Transformation of Family Law: State, Law, and Family in the United States and Western Europe.* Chicago: University of Chicago Press, 1989.

———. *Rights Talk: The Impoverishment of Political Discourse.* New York: Free Press, 1991.

Gomez, Carlos. *Regulating Death: Euthanasia and the Case of the Netherlands.* New York. Free Press, 1991.

Hendin, Herbert. "Seduced by Death: Doctors, Patients, and the Dutch Cure." *Issues in Law and Medicine* 10, no. 2 (Fall 1994): 123–68.

———. *Seduced by Death: Doctors, Patients, and the Dutch Cure.* New York: W. W. Norton, 1997.

Hobbes, Thomas. *Leviathan.* 1651. Reprint. Indianapolis: Bobbs-Merrill, 1958.

Jamison, Stephanie. *Assisted Suicide: A Decision-Making Guide for Health Professionals.* San Francisco: Jossey-Bass Publishers, 1998.

Jochemsen, Henk. "The Netherlands Experiment." In *Dignity and Dying.* Ed. John F. Kilner, Arlene B. Miller, and Edmund D. Pellegrino. Grand Rapids, Mich.: Eerdmans, 1996.

Jonas, Robert E., and John D. Gorby, trans. "West German Abortion Decision: A Contrast to Roe v. Wade?" *John Marshall Journal of Practice and Procedure* 9 (Spring 1976): 605–84.

Kamm, Frances, M. "Physician-Assisted Suicide, Euthanasia, and Intending Death." In *Physician-Assisted Suicide: Expanding the Debate.* Ed. M. P. Battin, R. Rhodes, and A. Silver. New York: Routledge, 1998.

Kant, Immanuel. *Lectures on Ethics.* Ed. Benjamin Nelson. New York: Harper & Row, 1963.

Keown, John, ed., *Euthanasia Examined: Ethical, Clinical, and Legal Perspectives.* Cambridge: Cambridge University Press, 1995.

———. "Euthanasia in the Netherlands: Sliding Down the Slippery Slope?" *Notre Dame Journal of Law, Ethics and Public Policy* 9, no. 2 (1995): 407–48.

Kevin Sampson v. State of Alaska (September 9, 1999). Reprint. *Issues in Law and Medicine* 15, no. 2 (Fall 1999): 199–219.

Kilner, John F., Arlene B. Miller, and Edmund D. Pellegrino, eds. *Dignity and Dying.* Grand Rapids, Mich.: Eerdmans, 1996.

Marzen, Thomas J., et al. "Suicide: A Constitutional Right?" *Duquesne Law Review* 24, no. 1 (1985): 12–42.

Mill, John Stuart. "Utilitarianism" and "On Liberty." In *The Philosophy of John Stuart Mill.* Ed. Marshall Cohen. New York: Random House, 1961.

Niebuhr, Reinhold. *Moral Man and Immoral Society.* New York: Scribner's Sons, 1932.

———. *The Nature and Destiny of Man II.* New York: Scribner's Sons, 1964.

Olafson, Frederick A., ed. *Society, Law, and Morality.* Englewood Cliffs, N.J.: Prentice-Hall, 1961.

Oregon Death with Dignity Act. Measure 16 (1994).

Oregon Revised Statues, 1996 Supplement 127.800–127.897.

Orr, Robert D. "The Physician-Assisted Suicide: Is It Ever Justified?" In *Suicide: A Christian Response.* Ed. T. J. Demy and G. P. Stewart. Grand Rapids, Mich.: Kregel, 1998.

Perlin, Seymour, ed. *A Handbook for the Study of Suicide.* New York: Oxford University Press, 1975.

Petrinovich, Lewis. *Living and Dying Well.* New York: Plenum Press, 1996.

Quill, Timothy. "Death and Dignity: A Case for Individualized Decision-Making." *New England Journal of Medicine* 324, no. 10 (March 7, 1991): 691–94.

Quill v. Vacco, 80 F. 3rd 716 (2nd Cir. 1996).

Reiser, Stanley J., William J. Curran, and Arthur J. Dyck, eds., *Ethics in Medicine.* Cambridge: MIT Press, 1977.

Reynolds, Charles. "Elements of a Decision Procedure for Christian Social Ethics." *Harvard Theological Review* 65, no. 4 (October 1972): 509–30.

Rodriguez v. British Columbia, 107 D.L.R. 4th 342 (1993).

Ross, W. D. *The Right and the Good*. Oxford: Oxford University Press, 1930.

Russell, Ruth. *Freedom to Die: Moral and Legal Aspects of Euthanasia*. New York: Human Sciences Press, 1975.

Sainsbury, Peter. "Community Psychiatry." In *A Handbook for the Study of Suicide*. Ed. Seymour Perlin. New York: Oxford University Press, 1975.

Spier, John. *Who Owns Our Bodies? Making Moral Choices in Health Care*. New York: Radcliffe Medical Press, 1977.

Stackhouse, Max. *Creeds, Society, and Human Rights: A Study in Three Cultures*. Grand Rapids, Mich.: Eerdmans, 1984.

Twycross, Robert G. "Where there is hope, there is life: a view from the hospice." In *Euthanasia Examined: Ethical, Clinical, and Legal Perspectives*. Ed. John Keown. Cambridge: Cambridge University Press, 1995.

Vacco v. Quill, 117 S.Ct. 2293 (1997).

Veatch, Robert M., ed. *Medical Ethics*. Boston: Jones and Bartlett Publishers, 1989.

Warren, Samuel D., and Louis D. Brandeis. "The Right to Privacy." *Harvard Law Review*, no. 4 (1890).

Washington v. Glucksberg, 117 S.Ct. 2258 (1997).

Washington Initiative for Death with Dignity, Washington Initiative No. 19 (1991).

Wolf, Susan. *Feminism and Bioethics: Beyond Reproduction*. New York: Oxford University Press, 1996.

Index